Urodynamics Illustrated

Urodynamics Illustrated

Edited by

Ranee Thakar
Philip Toozs-Hobson
Lucia Dolan

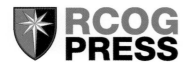

A machine-readable catalogue record for this publication is available from the British Library [www.bl.uk/catalogue/listings.html]

ISBN 978-1-906985-11-0

Published by the **RCOG Press** at the
Royal College of Obstetricians and Gynaecologists
27 Sussex Place, Regent's Park
London NW1 4RG

Registered Charity No. 213280
RCOG Press Editor: Jane Moody
Index: Liza Furnival, Medical Indexing Ltd.
Design & typesetting: Karl Harrington, FiSH Books, Enfield.
Printed in the UK by Latimer Trend & Co. Ltd, Estover Road, Plymouth PL6 7PL

Contents

About the authors   vii

Acknowledgements   xii

Glossary and abbreviations   xiii

Preface   xv

1   **Introduction**   1

2   **Setting up the equipment**   5
Lucy Swithinbank

3   **Flow rate testing**   21
Marcus Drake and Ahmed Shaban

4   **Cystometry**   35
Gordon Hosker and Joanne Townsend

5   **Videocystourethrography**   55
Sushma Srikrishna and Dudley Robinson

6   **Ambulatory urodynamic monitoring**   67
Kate Anders and Philip Toozs-Hobson

7   **Urodynamic artefacts**   81
Reeba Oliver and Ranee Thakar

8 Assessment of urethral function   **91**
J Robert Sherwin and Mark Slack

9 Bladder diaries   **99**
Matthew Parsons

10 Pad testing   **117**
Emmanuel Karantanis

11 Pre-test assessment using questionnaires   **123**
Ramandeep Basra, Nikki Cotterill, Swati Jha,
Conrnelius J Kelleher and Stephen Radley

12 Ultrasound as a tool in urodynamics   **135**
Demetri C Panayi and Vikram Khullar

Index   **141**

About the authors

Kate Anders RGN BSc
Lead Nurse, Urogynaecology
Ashford and St Peter's Hospital Trust
Chertsey
Surrey, UK

Ramandeep Basra MRCOG
Specialty Trainee in Obstetrics and Gynaecology
Addenbrooke's Hospital
University of Cambridge University Hospitals NHS Trust
Cambridge, UK

Nikki Cotterill PhD RN
Research Associate/Nurse
Bristol Urological Institute
Southmead Hospital
Bristol, UK

Lucia Dolan MD FRCOG
Consultant Gynaecologist and Subspecialist in Urogynaecology
Belfast Health and Social Care Trust
Department of Gynaecology
Belfast City Hospital
Belfast, UK

Marcus Drake MA(Cantab) DM(Oxon) FRCS(Urol)
Consultant Urologist
Bristol Urological Institute
Southmead Hospital
Bristol, UK

Gordon Hosker MPhil FIPEM
Consultant Clinical Scientist
The Warrell Unit
St Mary's Hospital
Manchester, UK

Swati Jha MD MRCOG
Consultant Obstetrician and Gynaecologist
Royal Hallamshire Hospital
Sheffield, UK

Emmanuel Karantanis PhD FRANZCOG CU
Senior Lecturer
School of Women's and Children's Health
University of New South Wales
Sydney, Australia

Cornelius J Kelleher MD FRCOG
Consultant Urogynaecologist
St Thomas' Hospital
London, UK

Vikram Khullar AKC MD MRCOG
Consultant Urogynaecologist
Imperial College London
London, UK

Reeba Oliver MRCOG
Subspecialty Trainee in Urogynaecology
Department of Obstetrics and Gynaecology
Croydon University Hospital
Croydon, UK

Demetri C Panayi MRCOG
Consultant Urogynaecologist
St Helier Hospital
Carshalton, UK

Matthew Parsons MD MRCOG
Consultant Obstetrician and Gynaecologist
Department of Urogynaecology
Birmingham Women's Hospital
Birmingham, UK

Stephen Radley FRCS(Ed) FRCOG
Consultant Urogynaecologist
Royal Hallamshire Hospital
Sheffield, UK

Dudley Robinson MD MRCOG
Consultant Obstetrician and Urogynaecologist
Department of Urogynaecology
King's College Hospital
London, UK

Ahmed Shaban MRCS(Eng)
Clinical Fellow in Urology
Bristol Urological Institute
Southmead Hospital
Bristol, UK

J Robert Sherwin MA(Cantab) PhD FRCOG
Consultant Obstetrician and Gynaecologist
The Whittington Hospital
London, UK

Mark Slack MMed FCOG(SA) FRCOG
Lead Consultant, Urogynaecology and Pelvic Reconstruction Surgery
Addenbrooke's Hospital
University of Cambridge University Hospitals NHS Trust
Cambridge, UK

Sushma Srikrishna MRCOG
Subspecialty Trainee in Urogynaecology
Department of Urogynaecology
King's College London School of Medicine
London, UK

Lucy Swithinbank MD
Director
Urodynamics Unit
Southmead Hospital
Bristol, UK

Ranee Thakar MD MRCOG
Consultant Urogynaecologist
Department of Obstetrics and Gynaecology
Croydon University Hospital
Croydon, UK

Philip Toozs-Hobson MD FRCOG
Consultant Urogynaecologist
Department of Obstetrics and Gynaecology
Birmingham Women's Hospital
Edgbaston
Birmingham, UK

Joanne Townsend RGN BA(Hons)
Team Leader, Continence Clinical Nurse Specialist
Oxfordshire Primary Care Trust
Oxford, UK

Acknowledgements

The authors are grateful for the assistance of Andrew Gammie, Clinical Scientist, Southmead Hospital, with the illustrations for chapter 2.

Glossary and abbreviations

ALPP	abdominal leak-point pressure
AUM	ambulatory urodynamic monitoring
ePAQ-PF	electronic personal assessment questionnaire: pelvic floor
Fr	French gauge
H_2O	water
ICS	International Continence Society
ICI	International Consultation on Incontinence
ICIQ	International Consultation on Incontinence modular questionnaire
KHQ	King's Health Questionnaire
LUTS	lower urinary tract symptoms
MID	minimal important difference
ml/s	millilitres per second
MHRA	Medicines and Healthcare products Regulatory Agency
NICE	National Institute for Health and Clinical Excellence
P_{abd}	abdominal pressure
P_{det}	detrusor pressure
P_{ura}	urethral pressure
P_{ves}	intravesical pressure
PVR	post-void residual urine volume

QALY	quality-adjusted life years: the arithmetic product of life expectancy and a measure of the remaining life years
Q_{max}	peak urine flow measurement (ml/second)
QoL	quality of life
UPP	urethral pressure profilometry
UPR	urethral pressure reflectometry
URP	urethral retro-resistance pressure
VCU	videocystourethrography

Preface

Ranee Thakar, Philip Toozs-Hobson
and Lucia Dolan

This book provides concise information to help clinicians who are new to urodynamics as well as acting as an aide memoire for established practitioners. It was born out of the recognised need for a manual that can be an instant reference for practitioners. The book follows many of the key principles taught on the joint Royal College of Obstetricians and Gynaecologists and British Society of Urogynaecology Urodynamics Course and uses the *Minimum Standards in Urodynamics* document and the International Continence Society standards as the main underpinning documentation for the text.[1,2]

We cannot overstate the importance of the expertise of the observer when attempting to obtain accurate and reliable measurements when performing urodynamics. Good urodynamic practice occurs when there is a clear urodynamic question, adequate patient preparation, appropriate technical expertise and an interactive test. In this book, we provide both a technical and clinical guide for the urodynamics observer through illustration of many of the practical steps and common clinical observations reported in the urodynamics laboratory. Several urodynamic investigations are discussed, ranging from the basic tests such as uroflowmetry and subtracted cystometry to the more complex namely videocystometry, ambulatory monitoring and urethral function tests. The key principles of measurement of physiological and pathophysiological parameters of lower urinary tract function are common, irrespective of type of investigation. This book should provide the core knowledge to undertake these measurements and an understanding of their limitations. Much of the information described for setting up equipment acts as a general guide when getting started and troubleshooting during investigation.

It is essential that these invasive, embarrassing tests are undertaken by clinicians who interpret the results in the context of symptoms rather than in isolation. The main learning points are summarised at the end of each chapter and guidance on avoidance of urodynamic pitfalls is provided within the chapter on artefacts. A selection of clinical cases has been included in many chapters to place the investigations within the context of a symptom complex. These examples and the core text should provide the key knowledge for everyday practice. However, it behoves us to say that true expertise will come from experiential learning and regular urodynamic practice. For the first time, the role and responsibilities of those undertaking urodynamics and those in training have been defined.[1]

Finally, we hope that you will keep this book in your urodynamics laboratory as an easy reference and, when you have outgrown its pages, that you will use it as an illustrative text for teaching others the fundamentals of good urodynamic practice.

References

1. Association for Continence Advice, British Association of Paediatric Urologists, British Association of Urological Nurses, British Association of Urological Surgeons, British Society of Urogynaecology, Chartered Society of Physiotherapists, Royal College of Nursing Continence Care Forum, United Kingdom Continence Society, Urogynaecology Nurse Specialists Network. *Joint Statement on Minimum Standards for Urodynamic Practice in the UK. Prepared by a working party.* UK Continence Society; 2009 [www.ukcs.uk.net].
2. Schäfer W, Abrams P, Liao L, Mattiasson A, Pesce F, Spangberg A, et al. Good urodynamic practices: uroflowmetry, filling, cystometry, and pressure-flow studies. *Neurourol Urodyn* 2002;21:261–74.

1 Introduction

The term 'urodynamics' encompasses a range of investigations which investigate the physiology and pathophysiology of the lower urinary tract. It may include one or all of the following:

- uroflowmetry
- standard cystourethrography
- videocystometry
- ambulatory monitoring
- urethral function tests
- pad tests.

Why perform urodynamics?

Urodynamic investigations are the cornerstone of understanding lower urinary tract symptoms. Historically, these investigations have been responsible for a seismic shift in our understanding of bladder physiology and pathophysiology, yet they remain controversial, simply because of the common failure to understand the basic principle of biological variation in the intermittent presentation of symptoms associated with pathology.

Urodynamic investigations are used to investigate bladder function and dysfunction in women with urinary symptoms, the most common being urinary incontinence. Guidance from the National Institute for Health and Clinical Excellence covers much of when investigations should be performed.[1] Broadly speaking, urodynamics is used when conservative therapies fail or when the woman has complex symptoms

1

or failed previous surgery. There are a number of tests available, each offering a different insight into lower urinary tract symptoms. However, exact protocols will be based on local service provision.

The first key principle is whether the test explained the symptoms. If it did not, is another test indicated? The second key principle is never to force the diagnosis. Referral should be based on local services as appropriate.

Performing urodynamic investigations

To obtain the most from the test, the practitioner must first recognise that urodynamics aims to reproduce pathophysiology in an extremely unphysiological environment. Women are often anxious and embarrassed when they attend for tests. Recognition of the artificial test conditions and the feelings of the woman are crucial to optimising the chances of reproducing symptoms. Patients must be treated with respect and the test should be performed in as private an environment as possible. Allowing adequate time so that the tests are not hurried is also important.

Before cystometry

Written information explaining the test should be provided with the appointment letter or when the woman attends the clinic. The information should include instructions on providing a urine sample in a sterile container, bladder chart and questionnaires and advice to come with a comfortably full bladder. Women who are using drugs to treat lower urinary tract dysfunction (such as anticholinergics) should normally stop using the medication for an appropriate period of time before the investigation. However, there may be occasional circumstances where the patient may be required to continue their medication when assessing the impact of an intervention.

If the woman is of childbearing age and is sexually active, there may be a need to carry out a pregnancy test before invasive urodynamics, to rule out a possible pregnancy.

Either verbal or written consent should be confirmed before commencing the test.

Reference

1. National Institute for Health and Clinical Excellence. *Implementation Advice. Urinary Incontinence: the Management of Urinary Incontinence in Women*. NICE Clinical Guideline No. 40. Clinical Guidance Implementation Tools. London: NICE; 2006 [http://guidance.nice.org.uk/CG40].

2 Setting up the equipment

Lucy Swithinbank

Introduction

Urodynamic equipment varies in complexity and a range of uro-dynamics machines is available. The choice of system depends on operator requirements. The Centre for Evidence-based Purchasing *Buyers' Guide Urodynamic Systems* may help to inform choice.[1]

The urodynamics laboratory

Guidelines have been published[2,3] and manufacturers normally provide training on any equipment purchased. The exact method of preparing equipment for a test varies. Calibration is generally best left to the service engineer or medical physics personnel and is usually under-taken as part of a service agreement.

Uroflowmetry equipment

Flowmeter

There are two commonly used types of flowmeter: the rotating disc and the weight transducer. The rotating disc can be dismantled for cleaning. A stand-alone flowmeter may be used separately from cystometry.

Commode

A commode with a funnel is placed above the flowmeter to enable accurate aim of the flow on to the flowmeter (Figure 2.1).

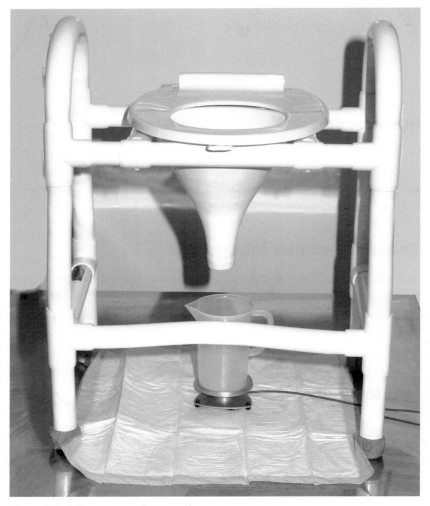

Figure 2.1 A flowmeter and commode

Subtracted cystometry equipment

There are three methods, depending on whether pressure is measured using fluid-filled, solid-state or air-filled catheters. The equipment used for each method is described below.

Fluid-filled system

The fluid-filled system is the currently preferred and most common method for cystometry.[3] External pressure transducers are mounted

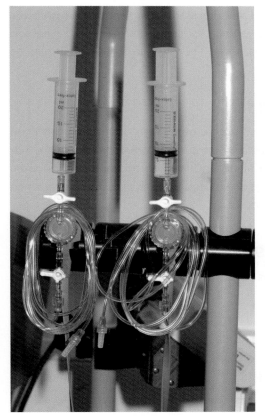

on the urodynamic equipment (Figure 2.2) and connected to the fluid-filled lines. The use of external transducers means that the system is prone to movement artefacts. The height of the transducers is adjusted when the patient's position changes relative to them. Fluid-filled lines are prone to air bubbles collecting during the test. Lines should be flushed to expel air when there is damping, which causes inaccurate measurement of pressure.

Figure 2.2 External pressure transducers mounted on the equipment

Types of fluid filled catheters

A fluid-filled pressure catheter is placed in the bladder to measure intravesical pressure and a second catheter is inserted into either the rectum or the vagina to measure intra-abdominal pressure. Either single-lumen or double-lumen fluid-filled catheters can be used to measure intravesical pressure.

SINGLE-LUMEN CATHETERS

If a single-lumen catheter is chosen, a second catheter called the 'filling catheter' is inserted transurethrally alongside the vesical pressure catheter. The filling catheter is used to fill the bladder with saline and should be 8 Fr or less in diameter. The pressure catheter should be 4.5 Fr or less in diameter.

DOUBLE-LUMEN CATHETERS

Double-lumen catheters have two lumens, with one lumen for filling with saline and one for measuring intravesical pressure. These are 6 or 8 Fr size and allow several filling and voiding cycles. Double-lumen catheters with smaller gauge are more prone to pump artefacts when faster filling speeds are used.

Abdominal (rectal/vaginal) catheters

Several makes of abdominal line (Figure 2.3) are available from manufacturers.

SOLID-STATE SYSTEM

A solid-state catheter-tip transducer is not connected to an external pressure transducer because it has a transducer mounted at the tip of the catheter.

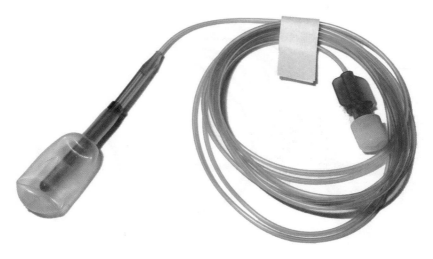

Figure 2.3 An abdominal catheter

A filling catheter, similar to that used with a fluid-filled system, is inserted alongside the solid-tip catheter and is necessary to infuse fluid. Solid-tip vesical catheters (Figure 2.4) can be either a single transducer or a double transducer, which can be mounted to measure urethral pressure simultaneously.

Solid-state catheters with a single-tip transducer inserted into the rectum and covered with a condom, sheath or gloved finger, can be used to measure intra-abdominal pressure.

AIR-FILLED CATHETERS

Air-filled catheters are disposable and have a valve that allows priming of the balloon and zeroing after catheterisation. Although they are commercially available, their use has not yet been validated.

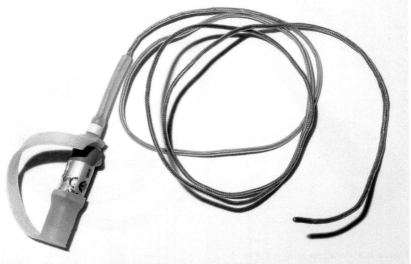

Figure 2.4 A vesical catheter with a solid-tip transducer

Other equipment

Manometer tubing can be supplied by the manufacturer. It is used to connect catheters to transducers. Transducer pressure dome covers vary depending on the machine. In a fluid-filled system, dome covers are required to transfer water pressure to the transducers and protect the transducers when the equipment is not in use. Three-way taps are placed both above and below the domes to allow for zeroing and flushing the lines during the test.[4] The Medicines and Healthcare products Regulatory Agency (MHRA) has recommended that dome covers, manometer tubing and syringes be changed between each patient to prevent cross-infection.[5] This is costly and time-consuming and so some trusts have introduced local rules concerning reuse.

Use latex-free disposables if a latex allergy is suspected.

Setting up uroflowmetry

The weight-transducer flowmeter is placed on the floor under the commode and switched on. The rotating disc flowmeter is assembled by placing the disc above the motor and is then switched on. The funnel is placed in the commode and the commode is placed over the flowmeter.

Enter the patient's details on the urodynamics machine then choose the uroflowmetry programme from the menu on the machine. Recording starts when a flow is sensed automatically or when a 'start' button is pressed. The user should check the settings on the machine.

Setting up subtracted dual-channel cystometry

Setting up can be considered as connecting the transducers and filling line and setting zero pressure. The technique for setting up will vary according to the type of system being used.

Connecting the transducers

FLUID-FILLED SYSTEM

Dome covers are 'primed' by flushing with sterile water. This can be achieved by either pushing fluid through using prefilled syringes distally or 'pulling' fluid through the dome from a distal giving set and bag using an empty syringe proximal to the dome.

A tap should be placed between the syringe and the dome, as placing the tap in the 'off' position to the dome during measurement prevents damping of pressures, which might otherwise occur.[5] The different positions in which the taps are placed are important for flushing, zeroing and recording (Figure 2.5).

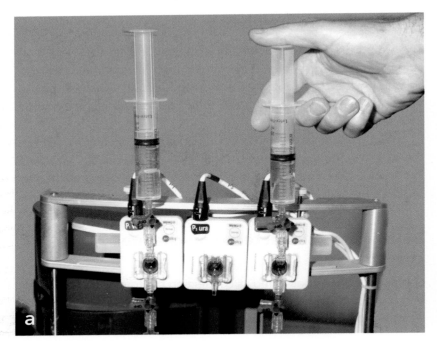

Figure 2.5a Three-way taps set for flushing

SOLID-STATE SYSTEM

Since the transducers are sited on the catheter tip, the catheter cables are connected directly to the urodynamics equipment.

AIR-FILLED CATHETERS

The interface cables should be connected to the urodynamics equipment. They should be left in the 'open' setting ready for connection to the catheters once inserted.

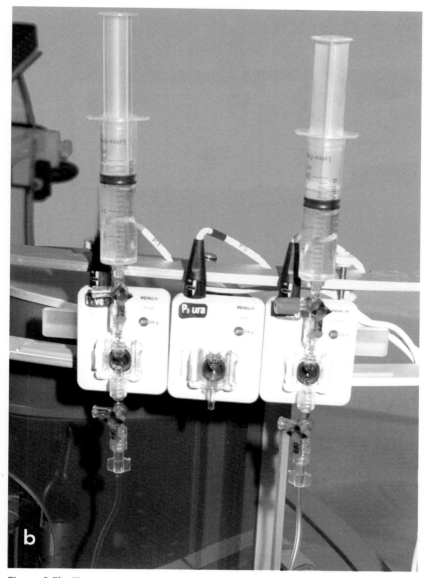

Figure 2.5b Three-way taps set for zeroing

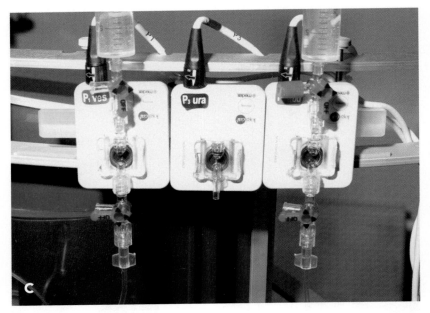

Figure 2.5c Three-way taps set for recording

Connecting the filling line

The filling line is connected to a bag of infusion fluid, usually 0.9% physiological saline, suspended from a weighted transducer using pump-specific tubing, depending on the equipment.

Setting zero pressure

The transducers are set to atmospheric pressure not to bladder or abdominal pressure. The method for zeroing is dependent on the choice of catheter (Figure 2.6).

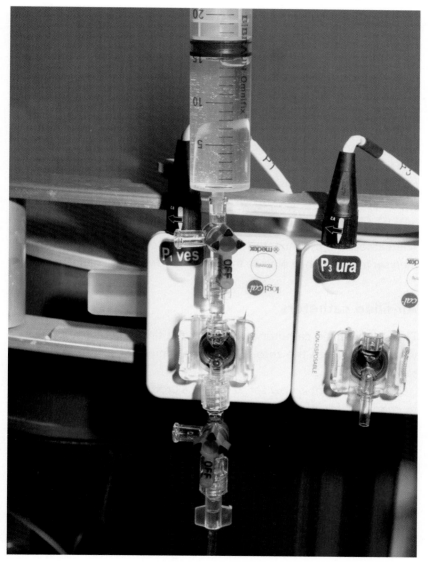

Figure 2.6 Zeroing the transducers to atmosphere with the taps open to atmosphere

FLUID-FILLED SYSTEM

When the selected programme has been chosen, the taps are turned so that they open to atmosphere. Press or select zero on the equipment.

The 'zero' of the machine can be checked at any time during the test by turning the tap so that it is open to atmosphere, if artefacts are suspected. Connect the catheters to the equipment.

After catheterisation, the catheters should be flushed through the dome once they have been connected to remove any air bubbles. The external transducers are placed at the height of the superior aspect of the symphysis pubis as the reference level during recording.

SOLID-STATE SYSTEM

The catheters are connected to the equipment after sterilisation and then set to 'zero' while outside the patient and while maintaining sterility.

Air-filled catheters

The only air-filled catheter available at the time of publication uses a valve that can set the zero outside the patient even after catheterisation.

The equipment is now set to record a urodynamic test. Please refer to chapter 7 for information on performing the test, including how to maintain quality and troubleshoot during the investigation.

Maintenance of calibration of equipment

Checking calibration

Calibration should be checked by users regularly. The timing of this procedure varies: every month is a good guide, unless there is concern about the accuracy of recorded measurements.

Checking calibration of the flowmeter

The flowmeter is calibrated using a constant-flow bottle. Water is poured into the flowmeter and the rate recorded and checked against the known constant flow rate. Alternatively, a recorded volume is checked by measuring the amount in the measuring jug against the volume recorded. This check is normally used instead of a constant-flow bottle.

Checking calibration of the urodynamic machine

FLUID-FILLED SYSTEM

Zero the transducers with the taps open to atmosphere then, with the taps set for recording a test, place the tubing ends at the level of the external transducers. The pressure should read zero (Figure 2.7). The ends of the tubing are raised to a height of 50 cm or 100 cm measured against a ruler or marker. If the machine is correctly calibrated, the pressures should also read 50 cm or 100 cm H_2O on the equipment (Figure 2.8).

SOLID-STATE CATHETER-TIP TRANSDUCERS

The calibration of solid-state catheter-tip transducers should also be checked regularly. This requires that the transducers are immersed to a set depth in water, rather than raised in air, or by means of a special calibration chamber which is capable of generating pressures in centimetres of water.

AIR-FILLED CATHETERS

Air-filled catheters are checked in the same way as solid-state catheter-tip transducers.

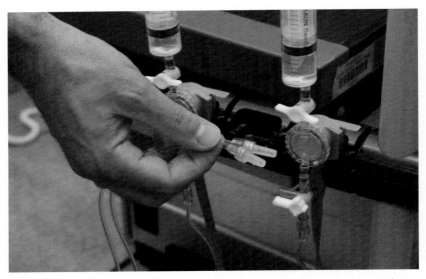

Figure 2.7 Checking zero with the tubing ends at the level of the external transducers

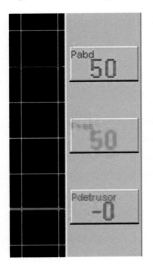

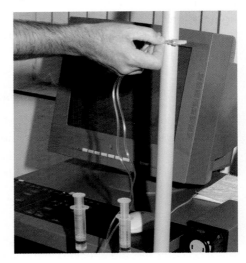

Figure 2.8 Machine correctly calibrated; manometer tube held at 50 cm H$_2$O on the equipment

LEARNING POINTS

- Pressure can be measured using fluid-filled, solid-state or air-filled catheters during subtracted cystometry. The use of air-filled catheters during cystometry has not been validated.
- Fluid-filled lines connected to external pressure transducers are prone to movement artefact.
- Solid-state catheters have a microtransducer in the catheter tip and are not connected to external pressure transducers.
- The MHRA recommends changing dome covers, manometry tubing and syringes between patients to prevent cross-infection.
- Calibration of the flowmeter can be checked by using a constant-flow bottle or checking the volume recorded after pouring a known volume into the measuring jug.
- Calibration of the urodynamics machine can be checked by raising tubing ends to a height of 50 cm above atmosphere, marked against a ruler, after zeroing the transducers to atmosphere.
- Transducers are zeroed to atmospheric pressure at the beginning of each test.

References

1. NHS Purchasing and Supply Agency Centre for Evidence-based Purchasing. *Buyers' Guide Urodynamic Systems*. CEP08045. London; 2008 [www.bui.ac.uk/Downloads/BuyersGuide.pdf].
2. Abrams P, Cardozo L, Fall M, Griffiths D, Rosier P, Ulmsten U, et al. The standardisation of terminology of lower urinary tract function: Report from the standardisation sub-committee of the International Continence Society. *Neurourol Urodyn* 2002;21:167–78.
3. Schäfer W, Abrams P, Liao L, Mattiasson A, Pesce F, Spangberg A, et al. Good urodynamic practices: uroflowmetry, filling cystometry, and pressure-flow studies. *Neurourol Urodyn* 2002;21:261–74.
4. Chu A. Dome set-up in urodynamics. *Neurourol Urodyn* 2007;26:594.
5. Medicines and Healthcare products Regulatory Agency. *The Reuse of Medical Devices Supplied for Single Use Only*. Device Bulletin DB2006(04). London: Department of Health; 2006 [www.mhra.gov.uk/Publications/Safetyguidance/DeviceBulletins/CON2024995].

3 Flow rate testing

Marcus Drake and Ahmed Shaban

Flow rate testing is a simple, non-invasive test, which can provide useful clinical information, although with important limitations. It is an assessment of the volume passed in unit time and is often undertaken in conjunction with other measurements, most notably post-void residual urine volume (PVR) measurement.

Methods of flow rate assessment

The two most common flow rate measurement systems are:

- **Gravimetric**: the weight of urine voided is measured over time; the flow rate is calculated from the rate of change in weight of urine.
- **Rotating disc**: as the urinary stream falls on to a spinning disc, it increases the weight of the disc, so the motor has to increase power to keep the disc spinning. The flow rate is proportionate to the power needed to keep the disc spinning at the same rate.

Both approaches are widely employed in current commercial systems. They are prone to variations in reliability and need to be calibrated before use. Regular checks are needed at intervals specified by the manufacturer and should also be done if the equipment is moved or disturbed.

Preparation for the test

Patients should have completed a pre-test frequency volume chart, which will show the typical and maximum voided volume. The set-up for uroflowmetry has been described in chapter 2. The flow rate machine should be in a private area. The patient should be well hydrated and prepared to wait for as long as needed to obtain an adequate result. The patient should be warned that the process can take some time. If they are in a rush to get somewhere else, representative flow rate results will be difficult to obtain.

Performing the test

Instruct the patient to void normally in their normal voiding position. Men should aim at the funnel and avoid squeezing the urethra or letting the stream 'wander'. Measure the PVR within 10 minutes of voiding. Two to three voids may be required because of intra-individual variability, which could affect the conclusions drawn.[1] Adequacy of voided volume should be assessed at the time, so that artefacts can be rectified.

What is assessed and how it is interpreted

Several parameters are evaluated with flow rate testing:

- voided volume
- maximum flow rate
- PVR (ultrasound or catheter).

Voided volume

Flow rate nomograms clearly show an effect of voided volume on flow rate.[2,3] At low voided volume, Q_{max} may be artefactually reduced.

Liverpool nomograms did not require a minimum voided volume.[2] Most clinicians recommend evaluating flow rate only above a voided volume of 150 ml. For men, a voided volume of at least 150 ml, combined with a threshold Q_{max} of 10 ml/s gives flow rate testing a positive predictive value for bladder outlet obstruction of 69%.

Above 550 ml, the bladder starts to overfill, causing artefactual reduction in Q_{max}. Some people can only void at high volumes; this should become clear when the frequency volume chart is examined. PVR is often elevated in such individuals.

Maximum flow rate

Normal ranges of maximum flow rate (Q_{max}) have been worked out by screening large populations of asymptomatic individuals. Q_{max} is affected by voided volume, so nomograms have been developed to aid interpretation:

- Liverpool nomograms[2]
- Siroky nomograms.[3]

In women, the normal Q_{max} is 20–36 ml/s, increasing by 5.6 ml/s/100 ml voided volume.[4]

Where Q_{max} is significantly below normal (usually taken as two standard deviations below the expected on a nomogram), there are several possible explanations:

- reduced bladder contractility
- low voided volume
- patient is inhibited (bashful voider)
- equipment has not recorded properly or been calibrated accurately
- bladder outlet obstruction.

Pattern of flow

The shape of the flow curve provides some hints as to the nature of a person's diagnosis. The normal curve should have a rapid upstroke, a curve with a clear Q_{max}, and decline quickly to end cleanly (see case 1, page 29). This is often described as 'bell shaped', although the trace is rarely symmetrical.

Abnormal patterns

Urethral stricture (men) Rapid upstroke; downstroke ends cleanly but Q_{max} is markedly reduced, giving a 'plateau' appearance (see case 2, page 29).

Straining Several peaks in Q_{max} caused by repeated Valsalva manoeuvres (see case 3, page 31).

Intermittent A poorly sustained detrusor contraction causes the stream to fluctuate. Appearance is similar to a straining pattern (and straining is often associated with patients with poor detrusor contraction).

'Supervoider' Very high Q_{max}; very rapid upstroke and downstroke. Not diagnostic but people with detrusor overactivity generally have flow rates at the top end of the range (see case 4, page 32).[5]

Artefacts Overestimates of Q_{max} owing to a high-speed squirt of urine from release of compression (Figure 3.1) or the stream 'wandering' on the spinning disc (Figure 3.2).

Attempts to measure objective parameters for describing flow patterns have been made.[5]

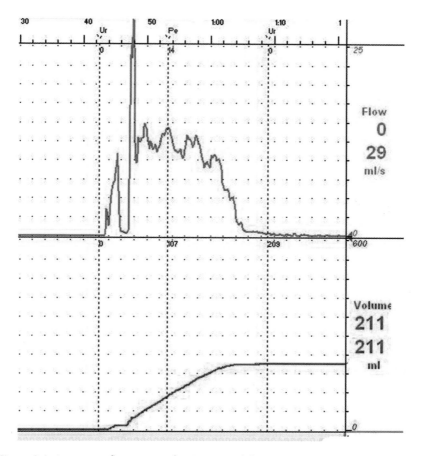

Figure 3.1 A common flow rate artefact in men with lower urinary tract symptoms. Shortly after start of voiding, the tip of the urethra has been held shut to build up pressure. Release then causes a sudden spurt, before the true voiding pattern re-establishes. The flow meter has recorded Q_{max} as 29 ml/second but examination of the trace quickly shows the artefactual nature of the recorded maximum and that the true value is nearer 13 ml/second

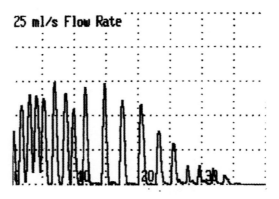

Figure 3.2 Intermittent stream resulting from a man allowing his urinary stream to wander over the collecting funnel; the voided volume was small and the trace unrepresentative

Women with incontinence

Low Q_{max} may be associated with voiding dysfunction after continence surgery or pelvic organ prolapse. A high PVR may occur infrequently after anticholinergic drug administration in overactive bladder syndrome.

Men with voiding symptoms

A low Q_{max} is not diagnostic for bladder outlet obstruction but it is a guide for the success of treatment and regular flow rate testing during follow-up can be a guide to recurrence (see case 1, page 29).

Patients with neurological disease

Interpretation is complicated by the greater range of possible pathologies. Suprapubic 'tapping' (banging the hand on to the suprapubic area, the shock of which can set off a short-lived bladder contraction, leading to partial emptying), is typically combined with straining (Figure 3.3).

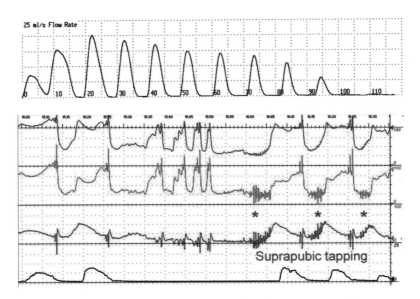

Figure 3.3 A young man with partial lumbar spinal cord injury. Top panel shows a highly interrupted flow pattern. In the lower panel, subsequent cystometry showed straining. The blue asterisks (labelled 'suprapubic tapping') show three occasions when he used banging on the suprapubic area to elicit a bladder contraction, causing expulsion of a little more urine each time

Low Q_{max} can also result from bladder outlet obstruction, with failure of relaxation of bladder neck, detrusor sphincter dyssynergia and outlet distortion (as in pelvic organ prolapse) possibilities, in addition to stricture or benign prostate enlargement.

Elevated PVR can occur in conjunction with detrusor overactivity, detrusor failure or bladder outlet obstruction.

(a)

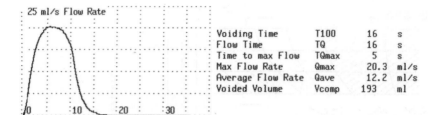

Voiding Time	T100	16	s
Flow Time	TQ	16	s
Time to max Flow	TQmax	5	s
Max Flow Rate	Qmax	20.3	ml/s
Average Flow Rate	Qave	12.2	ml/s
Voided Volume	Vcomp	193	ml

(b)

Voiding Time	T100	9	s
Flow Time	TQ	9	s
Time to max Flow	TQmax	3	s
Max Flow Rate	Qmax	3.4	ml/s
Average Flow Rate	Qave	1.9	ml/s
Voided Volume	Vcomp	17	ml

(c)

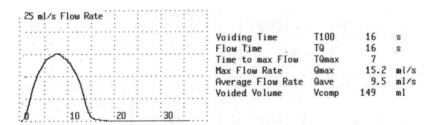

Voiding Time	T100	16	s
Flow Time	TQ	16	s
Time to max Flow	TQmax	7	
Max Flow Rate	Qmax	15.2	ml/s
Average Flow Rate	Qave	9.5	ml/s
Voided Volume	Vcomp	149	ml

Figure 3.4 Uroflowmetry traces showing: (a) a normal flow rate; (b) and (c) show that voided volume has a substantial effect on Q_{max} (case 1)

28

Clinical cases

CASE 1

70-year-old male with slight enlargement of prostate gland on clinical examination (Figure 3.4).

> Three uroflowmetry traces with different voided volumes are shown. Figure 3.4a shows a normal flow rate, with a rapid upstroke, good Q_{max} and slightly less rapid downstroke. In this man, there is only a low probability of bladder outlet obstruction. Three flows have been recorded for the same patient, with the top (Figure 3.4a) being entirely normal; the middle (Figure 3.4b) and lower traces (Figure 3.4c) show that voided volume has a substantial effect on Q_{max} and a reduction in Q_{max} can arise when voided volume is inadequate, even in the absence of bladder outlet obstruction.

CASE 2

Male with history of voiding difficulty presenting in acute urinary retention (Figure 3.5).

> Figure 3.5a shows voiding cystometry with stricture pattern flow rate, illustrating a normal upstroke, a plateau with reduced Q_{max} and a normal downstroke. This series also illustrates the use of flow rate testing to evaluate surgical outcome. The endoscopic pictures (Figure 3.5b) show stages in this man's urethrotomy, starting with the initial view of a tight stricture, with increasing depth of urethrotomy culminating in the final view seen in the bottom right endoscopic picture. The depth of scarring was severe, such that only scarring is still clearly apparent at the end

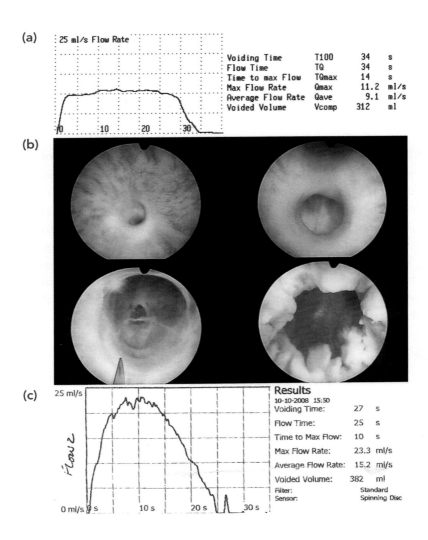

Figure 3.5 Voiding difficulty: (a) cystometry showing stricture pattern flow rate; (b) stages in urethrotomy, starting with the initial view of a tight stricture, with increasing depth of urethrotomy, culminating in the final view seen in the bottom right picture (c) flow rate pattern showing that urethrotomy has achieved a normal trace (case 2)

of the operation and recurrence appears a distinct possibility. The flow rate pattern in Figure 3.5c shows that urethrotomy has achieved a normal trace. Flow rate testing will be a valuable means of assessing recurrence during subsequent follow-up.

CASE 3

58-year-old female complaining of vaginal prolapse, slow intermittent urinary stream and recurrent urinary tract infections. Previous history of colposuspension (Figure 3.6).

The uroflowmetry shows an interrupted flow with several peaks in flow rate indicative of severe abdominal straining. A residual

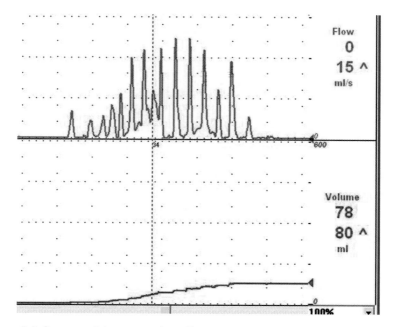

Figure 3.6 Severe straining pattern (case 3)

250 ml was drained with the filling catheter at onset of cysto-metry. Voiding cystometry confirmed a diagnosis of abdominal straining due to obstructive voiding, secondary to previous surgery and large enterocele.

CASE 4

52-year-old female with a history of frequency, urgency and occasional urge incontinence. No voiding difficulties (Figure 3.7).

This uroflowmetry shows a very rapid upstroke and downstroke with very high Q_{max}. This 'supervoider' was subsequently shown to have detrusor overactivity urodynamically.

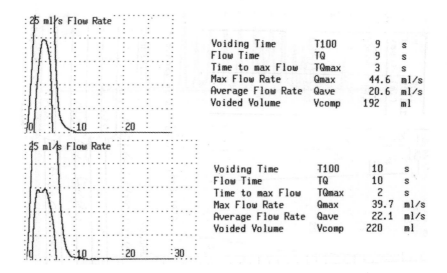

Voiding Time	T100	9	s
Flow Time	TQ	9	s
Time to max Flow	TQmax	3	s
Max Flow Rate	Qmax	44.6	ml/s
Average Flow Rate	Qave	20.6	ml/s
Voided Volume	Vcomp	192	ml

Voiding Time	T100	10	s
Flow Time	TQ	10	s
Time to max Flow	TQmax	2	s
Max Flow Rate	Qmax	39.7	ml/s
Average Flow Rate	Qave	22.1	ml/s
Voided Volume	Vcomp	220	ml

Figure 3.7 Uroflowmetry showing a 'super voider' (case 4)

LEARNING POINTS

■ There are two common types of flow rate system: gravimetric and rotating disc.

■ Information on typical and maximum voided volumes can be obtained from the pre-test frequency volume chart.

■ Intra-individual variation in flow rate may necessitate performing two or three voids.

■ Most clinicians assess flow rate when the voided volume exceeds 150 ml because of the risk of artefact at lower voided volumes.

■ Normal flow has a rapid upstroke and a 'bell-shaped' curve.

■ A plateau-shaped flow pattern is observed in the presence of a urethral stricture.

■ A residual of less than 100 ml is not regarded as clinically significant in asymptomatic patients.

References

1. Matzkin H, van der Zwaag R, Chen Y, Patterson LA, Braf Z, Soloway MS. How reliable is a single measurement of urinary flow in the diagnosis of obstruction in benign prostatic hyperplasia? *Br J Urol* 1993;72:181–6.
2. Haylen BT, Ashby D, Sutherst JR, Frazer MI, West CR. Maximum and average urine flow rates in normal male and female populations—the Liverpool nomograms. *Br J Urol* 1989;64:30–8.
3. Siroky MB, Olsson CA, Krane RJ. The flow rate nomogram: I. Development. *J Urol* 1979;122:665–8.
4. Jorgensen JB, Colstrup H, Frimodt-Moller C. Uroflow in women: an overview and suggestions for the future. *Int Urogynecol J Pelvic Floor Dysfunct* 1998;9:33–6.
5. Haylen BT, Parys BT, Anyaegbunam WI, Ashby D, West CR. Urine flow rates in male and female urodynamic patients compared with the Liverpool nomograms. *Br J Urol* 1990;65:483–7.

4 Cystometry

Gordon Hosker and Joanne Townsend

Introduction

Cystometry is the measurement of pressures inside the bladder both during the storage phase (before 'permission to void') and during the voiding phase (after 'permission to void') of urodynamics. Details of setting up the equipment for cystometry are described in chapter 2. Generic standards for subtracted dual channel cystometry can be found in the *Joint Statement on Minimum Standards for Urodynamic Practice in the UK*.[1]

Prior to conducting cystometry

Residual urine

Post-void residual urine is assessed immediately prior to cystometry by a dedicated bladder scanner, conventional ultrasound scanner or via inserting and draining the residual urine through the urethral filling catheter.

The advisability of draining the post-void residual urine before cystometry is controversial and many investigators choose to perform the cystometrogram on top of any post-void residual.[2]

Checking for urinary tract infection

Cystometry is usually postponed if the patient has a urinary tract infection because this could influence the urodynamic findings. Testing a specimen of urine with reagent strips for urinalysis with nitrites and leucocytes can provide a reasonable screening tool in the urodynamics clinic, having a sensitivity of at least 96.4% and a specificity of at least 88.5%.[3] If nitrites and leucocytes are present, there is a strong possibility of a urinary tract infection and the cystometrogram should not be carried out. A specimen of urine should be sent for microscopy and any infection found appropriately treated.

Starting the test

Lines are prepared and set up as previously described. The agreed reference for external transducers is the level of the superior border of the symphysis pubis.[4]

Baseline pressures

The values for abdominal pressure (p_{abd}), intravesical pressure (p_{ves}) and detrusor pressure (p_{det}) should be compared with the values shown in Table 4.1. The values of p_{abd} and p_{ves} will be at the lower end of the range if the patient is small and lying down and at the higher end of the range if the patient is large and standing up. If the values are outside these ranges then:

■ recheck set-up before continuing with the cystometrogram
■ ensure that the transducers are at the upper level of the symphysis pubis
■ zero to atmospheric pressure
■ check that the pressure lines have not slipped out of position.

If the problem persists, only proceed with the cystometrogram if you consider that you have a valid explanation for the baseline pressures being outside the expected range.

Table 4.1 International Continence Society recommendations for baseline pressures at onset of filling cystometry

	Pressure (cm H_2O)	
	Minimum	Maximum
P_{ves}	5	50
P_{abd}	5	50
P_{det}	−5	15

Checking for artefacts

Before commencing filling, ask the patient to cough to check that the pressure lines are recording intravesical and abdominal pressures correctly. Ideally, the strength of the cough should induce a pressure increase of about 100 cm H_2O. When the woman coughs, there should be an equal acute rise in both the abdominal and intravesical pressure traces. The detrusor pressure trace, which is derived by subtracting the abdominal pressure trace from the intravesical pressure trace, should show little movement (Figure 4.1).[2]

■ If the rise in intravesical pressure is smaller than the rise in abdominal pressure (Figure 4.2), this indicates a problem with the intravesical pressure recording (see chapter 7).
■ If the rise in intravesical pressure is greater than the rise in abdominal pressure (Figure 4.3), this indicates a problem with the abdominal pressure recording (see chapter 7).

A biphasic artefact on coughing in p_{det} (Figure 4.4) is caused by small physical differences in the two pressure lines that cause their respective transducers to respond at slightly different times to the impulse of the cough. Provided that the amplitude of the pressure rises in p_{abd} and p_{ves} are equivalent, there is no problem to correct and you can proceed to the next phase of the cystometrogram.

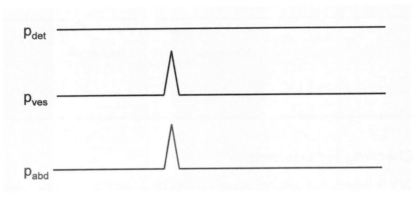

Figure 4.1 Coughing during the cystometrogram showing intravesical pressure (p_{ves}) and (p_{abd}) responding correctly

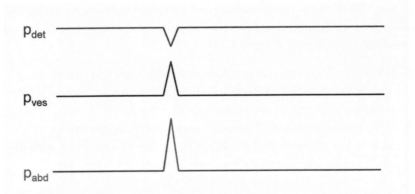

Figure 4.2 Coughing during the cystometrogram showing intravesical pressure (p_{ves}) not responding correctly

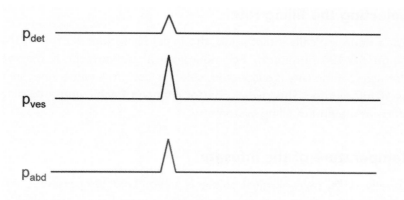

Figure 4.3 Coughing during the cystometrogram showing abdominal pressure (p_{abd}) not responding correctly

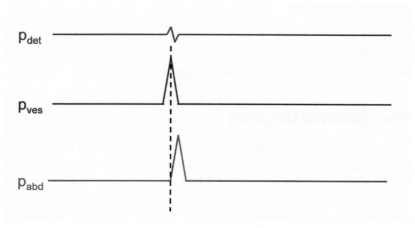

Figure 4.4 Biphasic artefact in abdominal pressure (p_{det}) arising from timing differences between the recording of intravesical pressure (p_{ves}) and abdominal pressure (p_{abd})

Selecting the filling rate

For a neurologically intact adult, the initial filling rate is often in the range 50–100 ml/minute. For neurological patients or if marked detrusor overactivity is suspected, select a less provocative rate, such as 10 ml/minute.[2] This gives a better chance of achieving a voiding study at the end of filling cystometry.

Temperature of the infusate

Usually 0.9% physiological saline is used. Low temperatures can artefactually induce detrusor overactivity, particularly at low bladder volumes. There is no evidence to show that body temperature should be preferred to room temperature. Make sure that the infusate has actually achieved at least normal room temperature (20°C) before instilling it into the patient.[2]

Patient position

Position can influence the outcome of cystometry.[5] The position adopted at the start of cystometry can be left to a combination of personal choice and the degree of mobility of the patient.

The cystometrogram

While undertaking bladder filling, the pressures are observed on the cystometrogram. All patient sensations should be annotated on the cystometrogram. Sensation may be classified as normal, increased, reduced or absent. The bladder diary provides a good idea of the patient's normal functional bladder capacity and is helpful in conducting the cystometrogram.[4] The International Continence Society has defined some of the sensations (Table 4.2).[6]

Table 4.2 Patient sensations as defined by the International Continence Society[6]

Sensation	Definition
First sensation of bladder filling	The feeling the patient has, during filling cystometry, when she first becomes aware of bladder filling
First desire to void	The feeling, during filling cystometry, that would lead the patient to pass urine at the next convenient moment but voiding can be delayed if necessary
Strong desire to void	The feeling, during filling cystometry, of a persistent desire to void without fear of leakage
Maximum cystometric capacity	The volume at which the patient feels that she can no longer delay micturition (i.e. has a strong desire to void)
Urgency	A sudden compelling desire to void during the cystometrogram (which should be recorded on the cystometrogram and noted if it reproduces the symptoms)

During bladder filling, the patient should be asked to cough every minute (Figure 4.5). If good subtraction is lost, the test should be stopped and the lines checked (see chapter 7). If the patient is sat over a flowmeter during cystometry, leakage will be recorded on the flow trace. If the urgency subsides, the operator may wish to continue filling, perhaps at a slower speed, depending on how much fluid is required in the bladder.

Normal detrusor function

When detrusor function is normal there is little or no change or contraction in p_{det} during bladder filling despite provocation (Figure 4.6). Table 4.3 shows some of the parameters of filling cystometry in a series of 72 women without any urinary dysfunction. This study suggests that the range of normal maximum cystometric capacity may be as large as 360–800 ml.

Bladder compliance is the relationship between change in volume in the bladder and change in pressure. Usually, compliance is calculated from the change in detrusor pressure from an empty bladder up to the cystometric capacity. Therefore, from the cystometrogram in Figure 4.6, p_{det} has risen from 0 cm H_2O to 4 cm H_2O as the bladder fills to 550 ml, which gives a compliance of 138 ml/cm H_2O.

Table 4.3 Cystometric parameters in asymptomatic women ($n = 72$) during filling cystometry; filled with 0.9% physiological saline at body temperature at a rate of 100 ml/minute

Parameter	Mean	SD	Minimum	Maximum
Age (years)	41.4	10.1	25	75
Parity	2.3	1.6	0	7
Residual urine (ml)	11	13	0	60
First desire to void (ml)	304	116	60	640
Maximum cystometric capacity (ml)	543	94	360	800
Compliance (ml/cm H_2O)	124	150	31	800

Abnormal detrusor function

Low (poor) compliance

Some bladders are 'stiffer' than others and do not have the same elasticity as normal bladders. For example, radiotherapy in the region of the bladder causes stiffening. Urodynamically, this manifests itself as a steep rise in detrusor (and intravesical) pressure during filling.

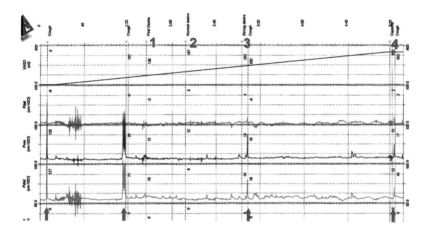

Figure 4.5 Cystometrogram with regular coughing (red arrows) to assess recording quality while the bladder is being filled at 100 ml/minute. The operator has recorded when the patient has a first desire to void (1), a normal desire to void (2), a strong desire to void (3) and maximum cystometric capacity (4)

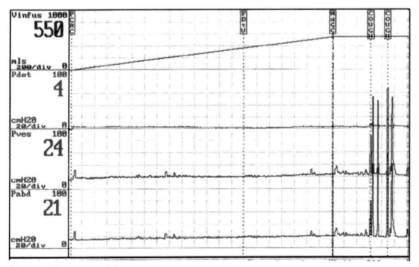

Figure 4.6 A normal filling cystometrogram

Typically, the value of compliance is less than 30 ml/cm H_2O and often associated with a reduced capacity. However, before a diagnosis of low compliance is made, filling is stopped. If the detrusor pressure remains abnormally high, the bladder is of low compliance. If the detrusor pressure drops to normal values when filling is stopped, then this is not low compliance, it is what might be termed poor accommodation (Figure 4.7), as some bladders need time to accommodate fluid filling them at nonphysiological rates.

High compliance

'High compliance' describes a large-capacity, 'floppy' bladder. Generally speaking, there is an underlying neurological cause. Typically, the value of compliance is considerably greater than 100 ml/cm H_2O and capacities of over 1 litre are not uncommon.

Detrusor overactivity

Detrusor overactivity describes involuntary detrusor contractions occurring during the filling phase of cystometry, which may be spontaneous or provoked. Phasic detrusor overactivity consists of waves of detrusor contractions seen during filling, which may or may not be associated with incontinence. Terminal detrusor overactivity is a single involuntary detrusor contraction occurring at cystometric capacity, which cannot be suppressed and results in incontinence, usually resulting in bladder emptying.[6]

There is no lower limit to the amplitude of an involuntary detrusor contraction but high-quality urodynamic technique is imperative to be able to interpret low pressure waves (less than 5 cm H_2O) correctly.

Not all detrusor contractions are of clinical significance. Work in asymptomatic volunteers shows that these contractions can exist without causing symptoms so you should record whether any

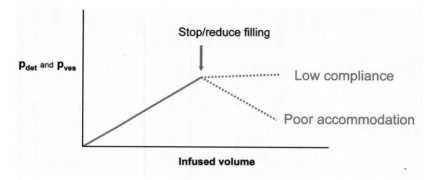

Figure 4.7 The difference between low compliance and 'poor accommodation'

contractions seen during cystometry are associated with events such as a change in the patients' bladder sensation (for example, first desire to void or urgency or whether there is any leakage). Modest detrusor contractions not associated with the patient's symptoms may be of no clinical significance.

Patient position, provocative manoeuvres and detrusor overactivity

If no detrusor overactivity is seen in the supine position, the patient should either sit up or stand up at cystometric capacity. The over-activity may only be seen if the patient is in a position other than supine (remember to relocate the transducers at the level of the symphysis pubis if the patient changes her position with fluid-filled lines).[5]

Other provocative manoeuvres to demonstrate or confirm the absence of detrusor overactivity include heel bouncing, jogging on the spot, listening to running water (Figure 4.8), washing hands under running water, coughing and refilling the bladder in a different position.

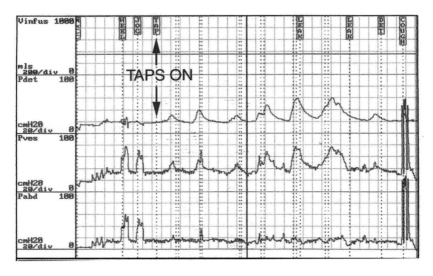

Figure 4.8 Detrusor overactivity provoked by listening to running water

Urodynamic stress incontinence

The International Continence Society defines urodynamic stress incontinence as urinary leakage seen during filling cystometry in the presence of raised abdominal pressure but in the absence of a detrusor contraction.[6] Leakage seen during coughing while the cystometric trace shows no evidence of a detrusor contraction confirms the diagnosis.

Coughing to demonstrate or confirm the absence of urodynamic stress incontinence is best performed with the patient standing or sitting on the commode. Other factors that induce the patient's symptoms, such as walking on the spot or shouting, may be employed to reproduce the reported symptoms.

If a separate filling line is used then it should generally be removed before testing for urodynamic stress incontinence. Additionally, any prolapse should be gently supported by, for example, a pessary, the blade of a speculum or a finger and the patient asked to cough again.

At the end of filling cystometry

It is usual to proceed to the voiding phase of urodynamics at this point. When the catheters are removed at the end of the voiding phase, the patient should be warned that they might experience some stinging during subsequent micturition. This sensation is common and usually lasts for a few hours and will resolve. Advising the patient to drink plenty of fluids may help to reduce the risk of developing a urinary tract infection. However, if these irritative symptoms persist for over 5 days, the patient should be instructed to take a specimen of urine to their general practitioner to check for a urinary tract infection.[7]

Clinical cases

CASE 1

59-year old woman with a history of radical hysterectomy and adjuvant radiotherapy for Stage 2a cervical carcinoma (Figure 4.9).

She complains of symptoms of urinary frequency, nocturia, urgency, urge incontinence and mild stress incontinence. Bladder diary indicates hourly voiding with average voided volumes of 100 ml and maximum volume of 200 ml. No history of urinary tract infection.

Filling has been stopped twice during the cystometrogram and on both of these occasions, as well as at cystometric capacity, the pressure has remained abnormally high, confirming low compliance. The maximum cystometric capacity is 218 ml and the detrusor pressure has risen to a value of about 65 cm H_2O, giving a compliance of 3.4 ml/cm H_2O.

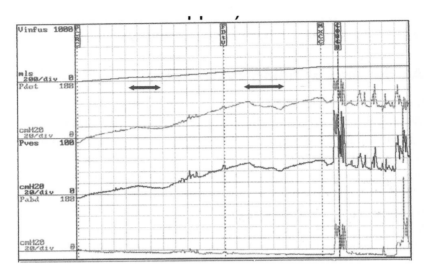

Figure 4.9 Low compliance; the arrows in red indicate periods when filling was stopped and the detrusor pressure remained elevated, thus confirming low compliance

CASE 2

Two patients each with overactive bladder symptoms (Figures 4.10 and 4.11).

In Figure 4.10, when urgency was labelled, there were rises in the red p_{det} trace. As these rises were also seen in the purple p_{ves} trace, this is evidence of phasic detrusor overactivity.

In Figure 4.11, marked detrusor overactivity is easily demonstrated on initial filling at 100 ml/minute. To ensure that sufficient fluid is in the bladder to study voiding, bladder filling is stopped at arrow 1, recommenced at a rate of 30 ml/minute at arrow 2, slowed further to 10 ml/minute at arrow 3 before stopping filling at arrow 4 (at a reduced capacity of 212 ml).

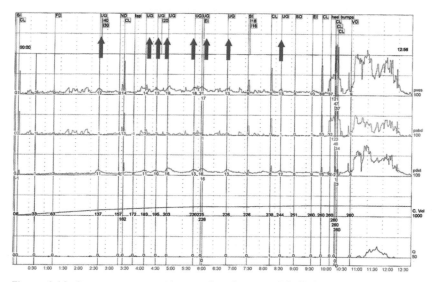

Figure 4.10 Cystometrogram with episodes of urgency labelled

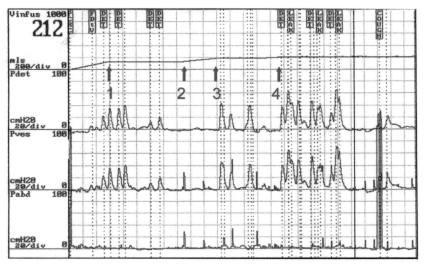

Figure 4.11 Reducing the filling rate when there is marked detrusor overactivity

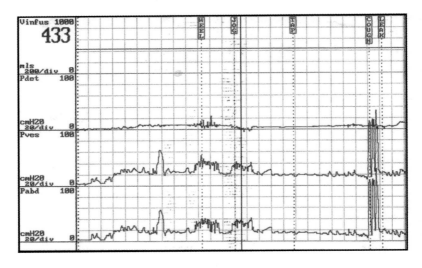

Figure 4.12 Urodynamic stress incontinence

CASE 3

53-year-old woman with symptoms of leakage of urine on coughing and sneezing. No urinary frequency, urgency or urge incontinence. No previous surgery (Figure 4.12).

Figure 4.12 shows a bladder which has a maximum cystometric capacity of 433 ml. It is stable throughout heel bouncing, jogging on the spot and listening to running water. The patient then coughs, which produces a strong increase in p_{abd} (red trace); this impinges on the bladder (p_{ves} – blue trace); there is no overactivity seen at this time (p_{det} – purple trace) but urinary leakage is observed: the patient has urodynamic stress incontinence.

CASE 4

47-year-old woman with symptoms of frequency, mild urgency, occasional urge incontinence and stress incontinence with coughing and bending (Figure 4.13).

At a cystometric capacity of 208 ml, the patient coughs, which produces a strong increase in p_{abd} (red trace), this impinges on the bladder (p_{ves} – blue trace) and provokes a detrusor

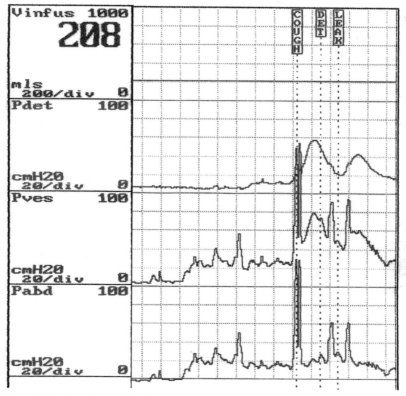

Figure 4.13 Cough-provoked detrusor overactivity

contraction (p_{det} – purple trace and p_{ves} – blue trace) and urinary leakage is observed: the patient has cough-provoked detrusor overactivity.

LEARNING POINTS

- Cystometry is usually deferred if the patient has a urinary tract infection.
- Baseline abdominal, intravesical and detrusor pressures should be within the normal range before commencing filling.
- Cough testing should cause an acute and equal rise in abdominal and intravesical pressures with little rise in detrusor pressure.
- Initial filling rate in a non-neurological patient is 50–100ml/minute.
- The infusate should have reached room temperature (20°C) before filling.
- Cough tests should be performed every minute during filling.
- Low compliance is typically less than 30 ml/cm H_2O and associated with low capacity.
- Detrusor overactivity is not defined by amplitude of detrusor contraction; however, modest detrusor contractions may not be of clinical significance in an asymptomatic patient.
- Urodynamic stress incontinence is the presence of leakage of urine with a rise in intra-abdominal pressure in the absence of a detrusor contraction.
- Provocative testing, such as a change of position or running water, should be used to elicit detrusor overactivity.

References

1. Association for Continence Advice, British Association of Paediatric Urologists, British Association of Urological Nurses, British Association of Urological Surgeons, British Society of Urogynaecology, Chartered Society of Physiotherapists, Royal College of Nursing Continence Care Forum, United Kingdom Continence Society, Urogynaecology Nurse Specialists Network. *Joint Statement on Minimum Standards*

for *Urodynamic Practice in the UK. Prepared by a working party.* UK Continence Society; 2009 [www.ukcs.uk.net].

2. Abrams P. *Urodynamics.* 3rd ed. London: Springer-Verlag; 2006.

3. Preston A, O'Donnell T, Phillips CA. Screening for urinary tract infections in a gynaecological setting: validity and cost-effectiveness of reagent strips. *Br J Biomed Sci* 1999;56:253–7.

4. Schafer W, Abrams P, Liao L, Mattiasson A, Pesce F, Spangberg A, et al. Good urodynamic practices: uroflowmetry, filling cystometry, and pressure-flow studies. *Neurourol Urodyn* 2002;21:261–74.

5. Al-Hayek S, Belal M, Abrams P. Does the patient's position influence the detection of detrusor overactivity? *Neurourol Urodyn* 2008;27:279–86.

6. Abrams P, Cardozo L, Fall M, Griffiths D, Rosier P, Ulmsten U, et al. The standardisation of terminology of lower urinary tract function: report from the Standardisation Sub-committee of the International Continence Society. *Neurourol Urodyn* 2002;21:167–78.

7. Bombieri L, Dance DA, Rienhardt GW, Waterfield A, Freeman RM. Urinary tract infection after urodynamic studies in women: incidence and natural history. *BJU Int* 1999;83:392–5.

5 Videocystourethrography

Sushma Srikrishna and Dudley Robinson

Introduction

Videocystourethrography (VCU), also known as videourodynamics, uses iodine-based contrast rather than 0.9% physiological saline, to allow simultaneous imaging of the lower urinary tract during urodynamic assessment (Figure 5.1).[1]

Equipment and facilities for VCU

The equipment needed for VCU is similar to that for conventional cystometry, described in chapters 2 and 4. In addition, it will be necessary to have a fluoroscopy unit with a high-resolution image intensifier and a tilt table (Figure 5.2).

Conducting VCU

Set-up, insertion of catheters and methods to reduce artefacts are similar to those for conventional cystometry, described in chapters 2 and 4. The bladder is filled with an X-ray contrast medium, such as isohexol (Omnapaque™, GE Healthcare). The patient may be either supine on an X-ray table or in a sitting position. At the end of filling, the filling catheter is removed and the X-ray table rotated so that the bladder can be imaged with the patient standing. Provocative manoeuvres are then performed.

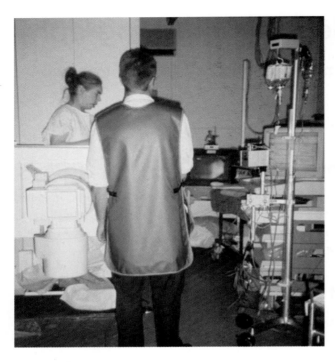

Figure 5.1
Videourodynamics

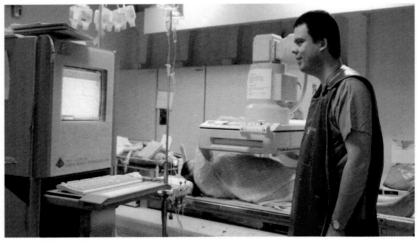

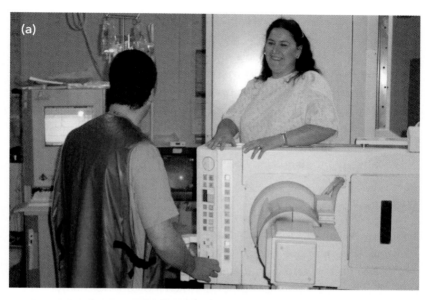

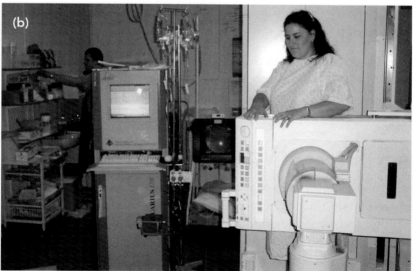

Figure 5.2 Provocation by (a) standing and (b) with running water

Urodynamic observations similar to those outlined in chapter 4 are recorded. It is the authors' practice to grade urodynamic stress incontinence as follows: leaking with the first cough is graded as severe incontinence, leaking during a series of three coughs as moderate leakage and leakage occurring only at the end of five coughs as mild incontinence; grading of incontinence may also be based on the actual quantity of urine lost.[2] If there is no demonstrable leakage during coughing and the patient's main complaint is incontinence, other provocative manoeuvres may be incorporated.

Voiding cystometry

The intravesical and rectal pressure recording lines are left in place, allowing simultaneous measurement of detrusor pressure together with the urine flow rate. Some women will subsequently have free flow rates and residual urine assessments which indicate normality.

Imaging

Fluoroscopic images can be obtained selectively during the filling and voiding study. The fluoroscopic images can be stored and reproduced individually or as continuous clips during key parts of the study. A recording can be made of the procedure for subsequent review.

Advantages of VCU

VCU allows accurate visualisation of the functional anatomy of the lower urinary tract. It is less sensitive in diagnosing detrusor over-activity[3] and those with refractory irritative symptoms may benefit from ambulatory urodynamic assessment, with its greater sensitivity in diagnosing detrusor overactivity.[4,5] VCU enables classification of urinary stress incontinence into four types (0–3), although this classification is

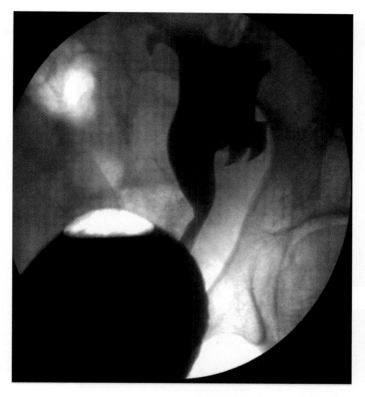

Figure 5.3 Neuropathic bladder with uninhibited detrusor contraction and associated reflux

no longer commonplace.[6] In patients with neurogenic bladder, VCU provides a more complete assessment (Figure 5.3), including identification of vesicoureteric reflux during filling or voiding phase and, in some patients, it may visualise detrusor sphincter dyssynergia. It will enable visualisation of anatomical abnormalities such as bladder or urethral diverticulae or fistulae (Figures 5.4 and 5.5) and bladder herniation (Figure 5.6). Although rare in women, it may allow identification of bladder outlet obstruction.

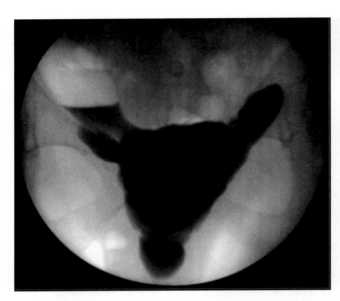

Figure 5.4
Multiple bladder
diverticulae

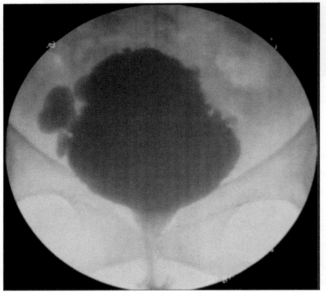

Figure 5.5
Multiple
diverticulae,
bladder
trabeculation and
an unprovoked
contraction with
leakage

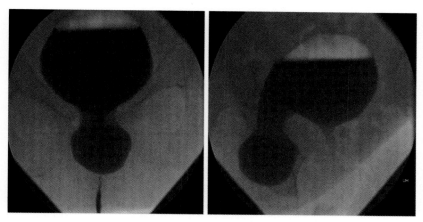

Figure 5.6 Bladder hernia

Limitations of VCU

Care with positioning is vital for optimal visualisation of the lower urinary tract. Visibility may be poor or absent with patients who are very obese. The requirement for radiation means that all clinicians should use radiation protection such as aprons and thyroid shields. The radiation equipment must be well maintained. VCU is costly but the cost may be justified by its utility in the management of complex problems. Anaphylactoid reaction is a recognised complication of intravenous administration of radiographic contrast media and remains a theoretical risk (less than 0.01%).[7]

Standardised terminology should be used to report results in keeping with the good urodynamic practice guidelines.[8]

Clinical cases

CASE 1

54-year-old woman with symptoms of vaginal prolapse, urgency, occasional urge incontinence and no stress incontinence (Figure 5.7).

Screening was undertaken selectively during provocative testing and at onset and end of voiding. The image shown was taken during cough testing upright after completion of filling. This shows radio opaque contrast in the bladder with loss of normal contour of bladder base owing to the presence of a cystocele (Figure 5.7). This image does not visualise the urethra, although no urodynamic stress incontinence was demonstrated.

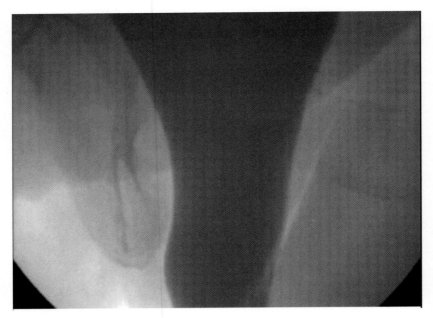

Figure 5.7 Large cystocele

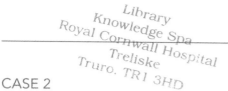

CASE 2

78-year-old woman with history of recurrent urinary tract infections, intermittent right loin pain, urinary frequency, nocturia and sensation of incomplete bladder emptying (Figure 5.8).

Screening was undertaken selectively during filling, on provocation and during voiding cystometry. The image shown was taken at the onset of voiding and demonstrates reflux of contrast medium into the right ureter and bladder diverticulae with 'fir tree' appearance of bladder contour owing to trabeculation. Voiding cystometry demonstrated Q_{max} of 8 ml/s with intermittent abdominal strain pattern flow and 150 ml residual.

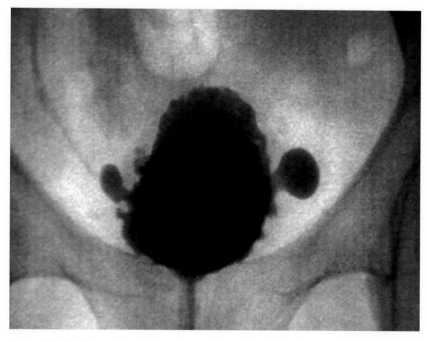

Figure 5.8 Bladder trabeculation, diverticulae and right-sided vesicoureteric reflux

CASE 3

49-year-old woman with stress-predominant mixed urinary incontinence. She has had a course of pelvic floor muscle training and a trial of anticholinergics (Figures 5.9 and 5.10).

> During filling cystometry the bladder remained stable. There was leakage, with coughing observed during imaging (Figure 5.9) in the absence of detrusor contractions. The urodynamic trace shows VCU correlation of mild urinary stress incontinence (Figure 5.10).

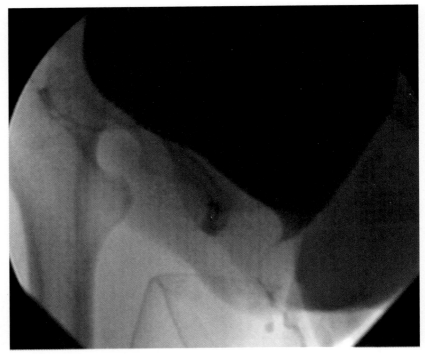

Figure 5.9 Leakage of urine during coughing at VCU

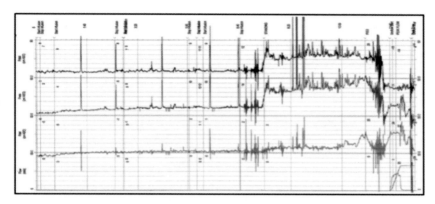

Figure 5.10 Urodynamic trace with VCU correlation of mild urinary stress incontinence

LEARNING POINTS

- Set-up, catheter insertion and methods to reduce artefacts are similar to conventional cystometry.
- An iodine-based contrast medium, such as isohexol, is used as the filling medium.
- Fluoroscopic images are obtained selectively during filling and voiding.
- VCU can be used to diagnose vesicoureteric reflux in patients with neurogenic bladder and to screen for anatomical urinary tract abnormalities.

References

1. Bates CP, Whiteside CG, Turner-Warwick R. Synchronous cine/pressure/flow cystography: a method of routine urodynamic investigation. *Br J Radiol* 1971;44:44–50.
2. Versi E, Cardozo LD Perineal pad weighing versus videographic analysis in genuine stress incontinence. *Br J Obstet Gynaecol* 1986;93:364–6.
3. Webb RJ, Ramsden PD, Neal DE. Ambulatory monitoring and electronic measurement of urinary leakage in the diagnosis of detrusor instability and incontinence. *Br J Urol* 1991;68:148–52.

4. Van Waalwijk van Doorn ESC, Remmers A, Janknegt RA. Extramural ambulatory urodynamic monitoring during natural filling and normal daily activities: evaluation of 100 patients. *J Urol* 1991;146:124–31.
5. Radley SC, Rosario DJ, Chapple CR, Farkas AG. Conventional and ambulatory urodynamic findings in women with symptoms suggestive of bladder overactivity. *J Urol* 2001;166:2253–8.
6. Blaivas JG, Olsson CA. Stress incontinence: classification and surgical approach. *J Urol* 1988;139:727–31.
7. Cartwright R, Cardozo L, Durling R. A retrospective review of a series of videourodynamic procedures, with respect to the risk of anaphylactoid reactions. *Neurourol Urodyn* 2008;27:559.
8. Schaefer W, Abrams P, Liao L, Mattiasson A, Pesce F, Spangberg A, et al. Good urodynamic practices: uroflowmetry, filling cystometry and pressure flow studies. *Neurourol Urodyn* 2002;21:261–74 [www.icsoffice.org/Documents/Documents.aspx?DocumentID=24].

6 Ambulatory urodynamic monitoring

Kate Anders and Philip Toozs-Hobson

Introduction

Conventional (laboratory) cystometry is the 'gold standard' in measuring bladder function. However, it is a static test and is considered 'nonphysiological', involving rapid retrograde filling of the bladder in a laboratory setting, which does not always allow reliable reproduction of symptoms. Ambulatory urodynamic monitoring (AUM), using micro-tip pressure transducers and a digital solid-state recorder, is a useful additional test for women in whom conventional urodynamics fails to reproduce or explain the lower urinary tract symptoms of which they complain. This system allows information to be recorded digitally, downloaded and reviewed at the end of the test. The trace can then be expanded or compressed without loss of information.

Differences between AUM and conventional cystometry

AUM is performed in accordance with the International Continence Society (ICS) *Standardisation of Ambulatory Urodynamic Monitoring*.[1] 'Ambulatory' refers to the nature of the urodynamic monitoring rather than the mobility of the subject and, although it records the same measurements as conventional urodynamics, it differs principally from conventional cystometry in the following ways:

- AUM is performed over a longer period of time (4 hours) and allows more than one cycle of bladder filling and voiding.
- It utilises natural bladder filling (a standard fluid intake, such as 200 ml half-hourly, is recommended).
- It takes place outside the urodynamics laboratory.
- Its portability allows reproduction of a patient's normal activities of daily living more easily. These may include manoeuvres designed specifically to identify the presence of involuntary detrusor or urethral activity or to provoke incontinence.

Indications for AUM

Indications for AUM are:

- lower urinary tract symptoms which conventional urodynamic investigation fails to reproduce or explain
- neurogenic lower urinary tract dysfunction
- evaluation of therapies for lower urinary tract dysfunction
- assessment of repeated pressure flows.

Performing the test

The care and observation of a patient undergoing AUM is as important in the diagnosis as the objective measurements and neither should be carried out in isolation. Checks on signal quality are highly important at the start, during the test and again before the test terminates.

Equipment

AUM systems have three main components:

- the recording unit
- the transducers
- the analysing system or software.

Recording unit

The recording unit must be lightweight and portable to allow freedom of movement (Figure 6.1). The memory, ideally, is digital, allowing compression and expansion of the trace. The recording unit must have

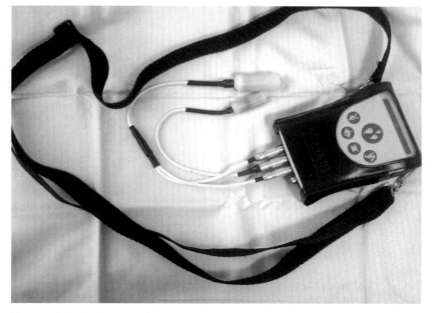

Figure 6.1 Ambulatory urodynamic monitoring equipment

AMBULATORY URODYNAMICS DIARY

Use the following codes in the diary below and remember to press the
event button when in the toilet. Please use the time displayed on
the front of the recorder.

U = Feeling like you want to/rushing to pass water
P = Passing water

T = Drinking tea or coffee
L = Leaking urine
W = Walking

S = Walking up stairs
D = Drinking any other drink, eg. orange, water.
C = Coughing
R = Sitting

DRINK A CUP OF FLUID AT LEAST EVERY HALF HOUR

Time	Event	Time	Event	Time	Event	Time	Event
09¹⁰	Start	11¹³	W	13⁰¹	walk		
09¹²	Walk	11²⁰	C/L	13¹⁰	cough leak		
09²²	D sit	11³³	sit	13¹³	Pass water		
09⁵¹	walk up. stairs L	11³⁷	Drink Tea	13²⁵	Walking		
09⁵⁹	P	11⁴³	U	13³⁰	urgency leak		
10¹⁰	W	11⁴⁶	P	13³⁴	Toilet		
10²³	R	12⁰¹	D				
10²⁵	D	12¹⁸	U				
10⁵²	urge P	12¹⁹	P				

Pressure lines are checked every hour. This will be done by Sister Anders.
Urogynaecology Unit, King's College Hospital

Figure 6.2 Patient bladder diary

a facility to mark events on the trace to allow better interpretation of the recording. This should be supplemented with a written or wireless patient diary (Figure 6.2). The recorder should have the ability to be connected to a flowmeter to allow simultaneous recording of pressure flow and an electronic pad to record simultaneous involuntary urine loss.

The transducers

Transducers are normally solid-state 7 Fr bladder and rectal catheters (Figure 6.3). Catheter-mounted microtip transducers allow greater mobility than fluid-filled transducers. They carry a greater risk of losing signal quality but there is less risk of movement artefact or changing reference point.

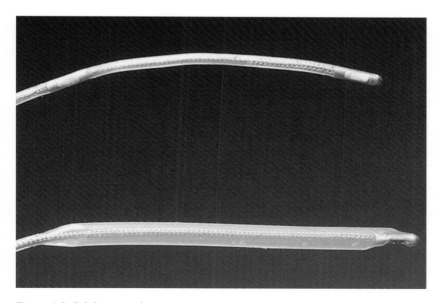

Figure 6.3 Solid-state catheters

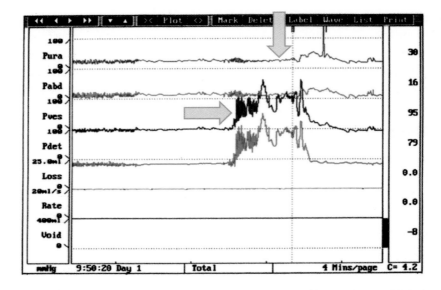

Figure 6.4 Rise in pressure recorded by one bladder transducer (pressure seen in lines marked 'Pves' and 'Pdet' but not in line marked 'Pura')

Microtip transducers should be calibrated before every investigation. All transducers must be 'zeroed' at atmospheric pressure before insertion. Most solid-state catheters have the pressure-sensitive membrane a few millimetres from the tip. Microtip transducers will record direct contact with any solid material as an apparent change in luminal pressure. It is possible to use a catheter with two transducers to minimise this artefact (Figure 6.4). Secure fixation of all catheters is essential.

Software

Figure 6.5 shows an example of AUM software ready to record.

Information for the patient at beginning of AUM

Patient compliance and straightforward but comprehensive instructions to patients are vital in obtaining a problem-free test. Information and possibly written instructions should be provided on:

- what to do in the event of catheter displacement or hardware failure
- how to complete and use a symptoms and activity diary
- how to use event markers
- the flowmeter
- the electronic pad.

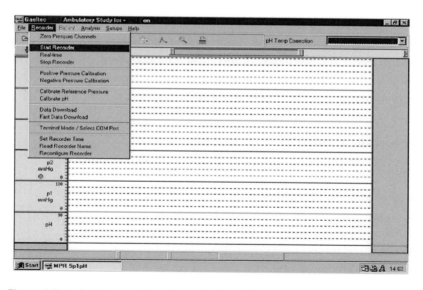

Figure 6.5 Ambulatory urodynamic monitoring software

Annotation of events during AUM

Information noted or recorded during AUM should include:

- initiation of voluntary voids
- cessation of voluntary voids
- episodes of urgency
- episodes of discomfort
- provocative manoeuvres
- time and volume of fluid intake
- time and volume of urinary leakage
- time of pad change.

Interpretation and analysis of results

At the end of the test, a real-time check on subtraction and the quality of the trace should be made. It is important for the patient to be present, as well as referring to the diary and event markers. Detrusor overactivity should only be diagnosed in association with urgency and/or urge incontinence; if two transducers were placed in the bladder then there should also be a detrusor pressure rise noted in both intravesical recordings (recorded as p_{ura} and p_{ves} on the trace).

The clinical report

The clinical report should include:

- the duration of recording
- description of signal and data quality
- fill rate, timing, method and volume of any retrograde fill
- dose and timing of any diuretics
- volume of fluid drunk
- number of voids
- total and range of voided volumes

- episodes of urgency, incontinence and pain
- detrusor activity (frequency, time, duration, amplitude, form)
- pressure and flow analysis
- results of provocative manoeuvres
- reason for early termination.

Troubleshooting

Constant vigilance, proper calibration, setting up and regular checks of the trace will minimise problems caused by recording measurements while not seeing a constant image. Rectal contraction and general interference can be difficult to avoid and they will not be obvious until the end of the test. Common problems and ways of minimising the risks are listed in Table 6.1.

Table 6.1 Common problems with AUM and suggestions for minimising the risk of occurrence

Potential problem	Minimising risk
Battery or hardware failure	Use new batteries Regular servicing of hardware
Loss of transducers	Careful fixation of catheters Instruction to patient to inform quickly if there is a loss of catheter
Abdominal interference, e.g. rectal contractions (Figure 6.6)	Insert transducer above sphincter; sometimes interference is unavoidable but a clear bowel at start of test will minimise this
Intravesical interference	Careful preparation and insertion of lines
Poor patient compliance	Comprehensive instruction and support
Lack of event marking	Comprehensive instruction
No flow data	Comprehensive instruction on how to use the flowmeter

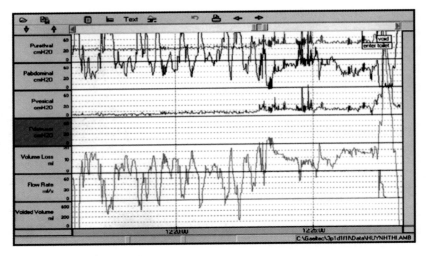

Figure 6.6 Rectal contractions

Advantages and disadvantages of AUM

Ambulatory monitoring in clinical practice has become more widely accepted, although controversy remains as to its usefulness in diagnosis and subsequent patient management.

Advantages

AUM has a role in monitoring voiding function. It has the ability to measure repeated pressure flows. Its advantage over conventional urodynamics lies predominantly in patient privacy during voiding. Conventional urodynamics, set up in the laboratory, often sees the 'inhibited or shy voider' and urinary flow data may be inaccurate or not obtained. AUM allows women to pass urine in a flowmeter in a private setting as and when they desire.

Disadvantages

AUM can be labour intensive and requires longer duration of testing, which limits the number of patients who can be investigated. There is a further learning time to become expert and it requires expensive and additional equipment to that used in conventional cystometry.

Clinical cases

CASE 1

32-year-old woman with occasional urgency and urge incontinence when out walking. Conventional urodynamics failed to demonstrate leakage. At AUM, phasic rise in the vesical and detrusor pressure associated with leakage on the electronic pad were observed during walking (Figure 6.7).

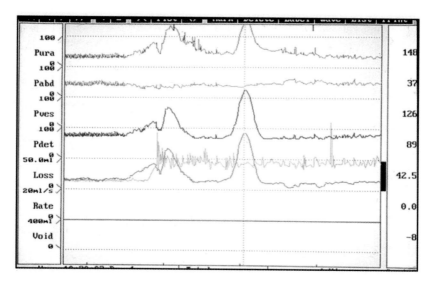

Figure 6.7 Detrusor overactivity with leakage

Detrusor overactivity (contractions on p_{ura}, p_{det}, p_{ves}) associated with leakage (elevation in the yellow line baseline) was diagnosed.

CASE 2

45-year old woman who had a transvaginal tape procedure complained of symptoms of stress incontinence when jogging. Conventional cystometry failed to demonstrate urinary stress incontinence.

The woman was instructed to include a gentle jog in the park while wearing the ambulatory monitoring device. Leakage in the absence of a detrusor contraction was observed with rises in intra-abdominal pressure during jogging (Figure 6.8) marked on the record of events.

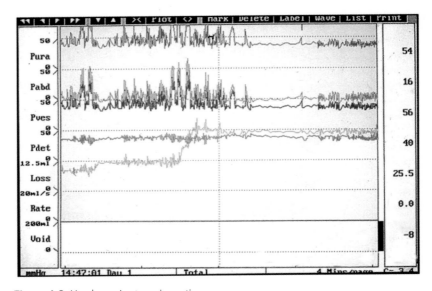

Figure 6.8 Urodynamic stress incontinence

LEARNING POINTS

■ Ambulatory urodynamics is usually undertaken over a 4-hour period, thereby incorporating more than one filling and voiding cycle.

■ AUM is undertaken outside the laboratory to mimic the activities of normal daily living.

■ Attention to proper calibration and patient ability to follow clear written and verbal instructions are vital in achieving a problem-free test.

■ Indications for AUM include failure to reproduce symptoms with conventional tests, neurogenic lower urinary tract dysfunction and repeated flow testing.

■ 7 Fr solid-state microtip transducers are commonly used as pressure transducers.

■ Common problems encountered include loss of catheters, abdominal and vesical interference, failure to record events or flow and poor patient compliance.

Reference

1. van Waalwick van Doorn E, Anders K, Khullar V, Kulseng-Hanssen S, Pesce F, Robertson A, et al. Standardisation of Ambulatory Urodynamic Reporting: Report of the Standardisation Sub-committee of the International Continence Society for Ambulatory Urodynamic Studies. *Neurourol Urodyn* 2000;19:113–25.

7 Urodynamic artefacts

Reeba Oliver and Ranee Thakar

Introduction

Data quality and documentation of variance are key for urodynamics studies to be valid and symptoms must be reproduced to be able to make a diagnosis. Accurate reporting requires knowledge of pathophysiological parameters and the ability to detect artefacts. If inaccuracies are discovered, they should be corrected contemporaneously.

Spurious and inaccurate observations are known as artefacts. These occur because of pitfalls including:

- failure to reproduce symptoms
- observations normally indicating pathology occurring in the absence of disease
- biological variability leading to false negatives
- the wide variation within the physiological range of the normal population.

Factors affecting urodynamic investigations

Several factors may influence the measurements recorded on the cystometrogram:

- filling medium type, temperature and rate of infusion
- catheter size
- patient position

- artificial environment
- communication
- inaccuracies in uroflowmetry
- equipment (all equipment should conform to International Continence Society technical specifications)
- voided volumes less than 150–200 ml.

Uroflowmetry artefacts

Artefacts during uroflowmetry may arise owing to several factors, which can be broadly classified into two groups: extracorporeal and intracorporeal.

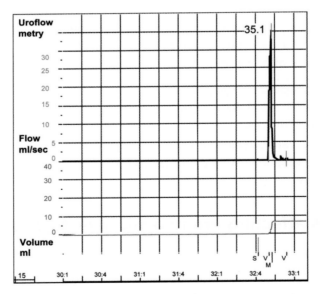

Figure 7.1 Uroflowmetry trace demonstrating changes owing to patient movement. The abrupt spike is recorded by the machine as the maximum flow rate (35.1 ml/s). This is an artefact and gives a falsely high maximum flow rate. The actual maximum flow rate should be read as in the region of 20 ml/s

Extracorporeal causes include:

■ flow interference between the collecting funnel and flowmeter
■ movement of the stream across the funnel surface
■ patient movement (Figure 7.1).

Intracorporeal causes include:

■ rapid abdominal straining (Figure 7.2)
■ fast and rapid flow (Figure 7.3).

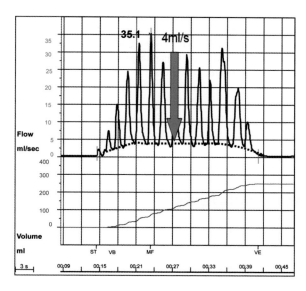

Figure 7.2 Changes in uroflowmetry recording induced by rapid abdominal straining. The solid arrow on the curve drawn denotes manually read maximum flow rate. Although the computerised reading shows 35.1 ml/s, manual assessment of flow using smoothed curve denoted the actual flow rate of 4 ml/s

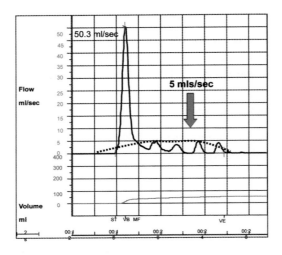

Figure 7.3 Changes in uroflowmetry recording induced by fast and rapid flow; solid arrow on the curve drawn denotes manually read maximum flow rate. Although the computerised reading shows 50.3 ml/s, manual assessment of flow using smoothed curve denoted the actual flow rate of 5 ml/s

Recommendations to minimise uroflowmetry artefacts include ensuring privacy, checking the report and tracing immediately, correcting artefacts manually and checking that the void was representative of normal.

Cystometry artefacts

The setting up of equipment at the beginning of cystometry has been described in chapters 2 and 4.

Common causes which lead to erroneous observations on the cystometrogram include:

- failure to set zero pressure correctly to atmosphere at the beginning of the test, with the transducers at the level of the upper border of the patient's symphysis pubis (Figure 7.4)

- impairment of p_{abd} transmission (Figure 7.5) owing to:
  - ☐ faecal loading impairing pressure transmission
  - ☐ damping from air in fluid-filled catheters
  - ☐ contact of the balloon with the wall of the rectum
- impairment of p_{ves} transmission (Figure 7.6) owing to:
  - ☐ catheter not located in the bladder
  - ☐ catheter blocked or kinked
  - ☐ catheter touching the bladder wall
  - ☐ catheter not disconnected from filling line when piggybacked
- change in p_{ves} or p_{abd} owing to movement or disconnection of a catheter (Figure 7.7)
- gradual rise in p_{ves} owing to the pressure catheter migrating into the bladder neck region (Figure 7.8)
- physiological artefacts, such as rectal contractions: mirroring in the p_{det} (Figure 7.9)
- baseline drift caused by an air bubble in a fluid-filled line or hysteresis artefact in solid state transducer.

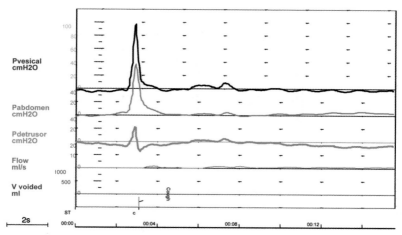

Figure 7.4 Cystometry recording showing incorrect zero pressure caused by setting the catheter-mounted pressure transducers to zero following, rather than prior to insertion in the body

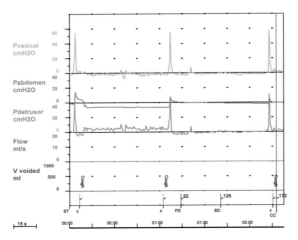

Figure 7.5 Cystometry recording showing impairment of abdominal pressure transmission to the transducer as evidenced by lack of signal response in p_{abd} trace. If abdominal pressure transmission to the transducer is impaired, flush the catheters with water and, if this fails, replace the catheters

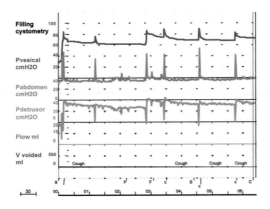

Figure 7.6 Cystometry recording showing impairment of intravesical pressure transmission to the transducer as evidenced by lack of signal response in p_{ves} trace. If intravesical pressure transmission to the transducer is impaired, flush the p_{ves} line (maximum 10 ml) slowly, add fluid to the bladder via filling lumen and check catheter position and reposition if necessary

86

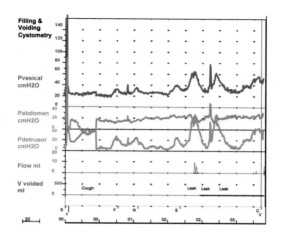

Figure 7.7 Cystometry recording showing if a sudden drop in p_{abd}. If a sudden drop or increase in p_{ves} or p_{abd} occurs ensure that the pressure catheters have not been displaced from the bladder or rectum and reposition them as required

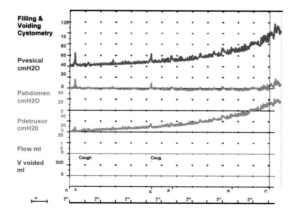

Figure 7.8 Cystometry recording showing a gradual rise in p_{ves}. If gradual rise in p_{ves} occurs, assess by asking the patient to cough to ensure correct transmission and stop or slow bladder filling if pressure rise is related to fast fill

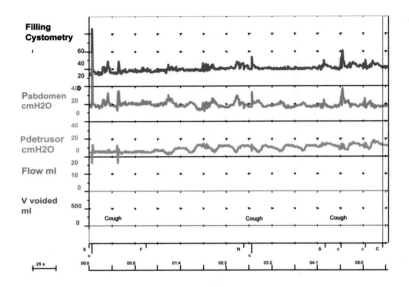

Figure 7.9 Cystometry recording showing rectal contractions. Rectal contractions are seen frequently and defined as multiple fluctuations in abdominal pressure of at least 5 cm H_2O. The clinician must recognise the contractions and not allow them to interfere with the interpretation of the bladder function study

Recommendations to minimise artefacts

Initial quality checks will prevent the majority of artefacts. Rectify problems with the signal at the beginning of the test and check continuously during the test.

Perform a cough test intermittently during the study. If cough spikes are lost, establish the cause and correct immediately. The p_{abd} and p_{ves} recordings are 'live', showing minor variations of breathing or talking which should not appear in p_{det}.

Pressure flow artefacts

Artefacts may arise during the voiding phase owing to displacement of the vesical or rectal pressure transducer or inadequate pressure transmission (Figure 7.10).

Recommendations to minimise pressure flow artefacts

Cough before and after voiding.

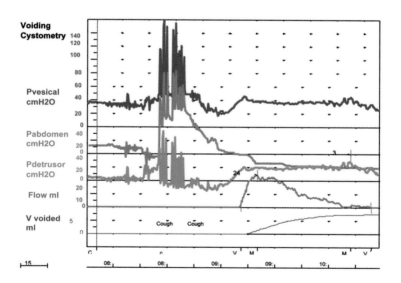

Figure 7.10 Pressure flow recording showing displacement of the rectal pressure transducer. Coughs immediately before and after voiding should be included in the study to ensure that the vesical and rectal pressure transducers are in place

LEARNING POINTS

- Artefacts are spurious and inaccurate urodynamic observations.
- Artefacts arise owing to physical properties of infusant and catheters, patient positioning, artificial environment or technical inaccuracies with recording pressures.
- Artefacts at uroflowmetry are minimised by checking calibration regularly and asking the patient to void normally in private.
- Artefacts during cystometry can be minimised by zeroing transducers to atmospheric pressure, expelling air bubbles and checking for good subtraction with cough testing before filling, at 1-minute intervals during filling and before and after voiding.
- Abdominal and intravesical pressures should show minor 'live' variations during filling which do not appear in the detrusor pressure recording.

8 Assessment of urethral function

J Robert Sherwin and Mark Slack

Introduction

Many tests of urethral function have been proposed and the International Continence Society (ICS) has suggested standardisation of the performance of some of these studies and has defined parameters for measurements.[1] Components of the urethral continence mechanism (Figure 8.1) are the submucosal vasculature, the urethral smooth muscle, the urethral striated sphincter, the bladder neck and the urethral supports. Failure of one or more of these structures can result in incontinence.

Urethral function tests during filling cystometry

Two tests may be included to assess urethral function specifically during filling cystometry:

- vesical or detrusor leak-point pressure estimation
- abdominal leak-point pressure (ALPP).

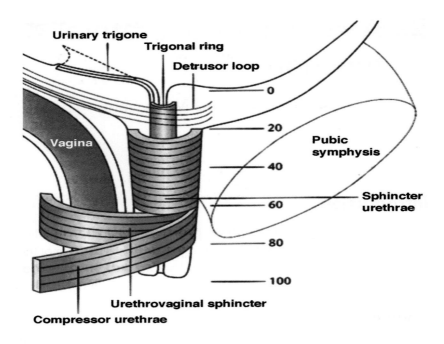

Figure 8.1 Anatomy of the female urethral sphincter

Vesical or detrusor leak-point pressure

Vesical or detrusor leak-point pressure is recorded as the detrusor pressure at the instance of leakage and is considered to be an indirect measure of urethral resistance.[2]

ALPP

ALPP measures the vesical pressure at which leakage occurs during gradual increase in intra-abdominal pressure in the absence of detrusor overactivity. Patients are instructed to produce a graded Valsalva, thereby increasing intra-abdominal pressure while in the upright position at a bladder volume of 250 ml and after reduction of pelvic organ prolapse.

Urethral function during voiding cystometry

Tests of urethral function during voiding cystometry measure the relationship between pressure in the bladder and urine flow rate.[1] Increased detrusor pressure and synchronous, reduced urine flow rates may indicate 'abnormal urethral function'. This may be caused by anatomical abnormalities such as a urethral stricture or urethral over activity.

Tests of urethral function

Additional tests to assess urethral function specifically may be included when more detailed information on urethral function is desirable.

Urethral pressure profilometry

Urethral pressure profilometry (UPP) provides a graph indicating the intraluminal pressure along the length of the urethra (Figure 8.2).[2] A water-perfused catheter, pressure-tip transducer, balloon catheter or air-filled catheter may be used. Profilometry may be performed at rest, during voiding or as a stress test (coughing, straining or Valsalva). The patient positioning is supine (upright position increases maximum urethral closure pressure), at no specified bladder volume and with pelvic organ prolapse reduced. The test is repeated three to six times, for reproducibility.

The parameters recorded are:

- absolute urethral length
- functional urethral length
- maximum urethral pressure
- maximum urethral closure pressure.

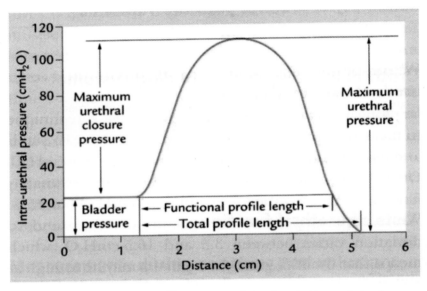

Figure 8.2 Urethral pressure profile parameters (reproduced with permission from Informa Healthcare)

Urethral retro-resistance pressure

Urethral retro-resistance pressure (URP) has been defined as the pressure required to achieve and maintain an open urethral sphincter.[3]

Urethral pressure reflectometry

Urethral pressure reflectometry (UPR) is measured using a 5-mm diameter polyurethane bag and urethral transducer. Urethral pressure and urethral cross-sectional area are simultaneously measured along the entire length of the urethra.[4] Initial studies have compared UPR with UPP and show a close correlation with maximum urethral closure pressure measurements, with better reproducibility for URP.[4]

Indications for urethral function tests

Controversy remains as to the validity and utility of urethral function tests. They are most often used in combination with other urodynamic tests or in a research protocol. There are no absolute indications for these tests in normal clinical practice.

Tests of urethral function may be applied in some clinical circumstances. They may be useful to identify patients with idiopathic voiding dysfunction or idiopathic urinary retention. If urethral instability is suspected, continuous urethral pressure recording, which measures urethral pressure at one point along the urethra for a fixed period of time, is helpful. Tests of urethral function may also be useful in identifying incompetent urethral closure mechanisms before obstructive surgery for stress urinary incontinence. A maximum urethral closure pressure of less than 20 cm H_2O may be associated with a higher surgical failure rate.

Potential advantages of urethral function tests

- Balloon catheters measure a true hydrostatic pressure and average out variations in pressure over the length of the balloon; pressure-tip transducers measure rapid changes in pressure.[5]
- An ALPP of less than 60 cm H_2O has been proposed as an indicator of incompetent urethral closure mechanism, although its role in the prediction of outcome is controversial.[6]

Limitations of urethral function tests

- Micro-tip transducers are fragile and expensive and depend upon transducer orientation.
- Tests of urethral function have low test reproducibility.
- The introduction of a urethral catheter may prevent the urethra functioning normally, leading to aberrant readings; for example,

urethral pressure is defined as the fluid pressure needed to just open a closed urethra.

■ No reference values have been identified to enable differentiation of normal, stress urinary incontinence or detrusor overactivity.

■ Successful surgical treatment for stress urinary incontinence does not correlate with changes in UPP parameters.

Summary

Currently available methods of assessing urethral pressure have significant limitations and their routine use is not recommended. For a small number of patients, where urethral pathology is suspected, judicious use of UPP may inform and aid diagnosis.

LEARNING POINTS
■ The role of specific tests for urethral function is controversial.

■ Urethral pressure profilometry is the most commonly used test of urethral function. It produces a graph of intraluminal pressure along the length of the urethra.

■ Poor reproducibility and wide variation within a normal population limits useful application within clinical practice.

References

1. Lose G, Griffiths D, Hosker G, Kulseng-Hanssen S, Perucchini D, Schafer W, et al. Standardisation of urethral pressure measurement: report from the Standardisation Sub-Committee of the International Continence Society. *Neurourol Urodyn* 2002;21:258–60.
2. Wan J, McGuire EJ, Bloom DA, Ritchey ML. Stress leak point pressure: a diagnostic tool for incontinent children. *J Urol* 1993;150:700–2.
3. Slack M, Culligan P, Tracey M, Hunsicker K, Patel B, Sumeray M. Relationship of urethral retro-resistance pressure to urodynamic measurements and incontinence severity. *Neurourol Urodyn* 2004;23:109–14.

4. Klarskov N, Lose G. Urethral pressure reflectometry; a novel technique for simultaneous recording of pressure and cross-sectional area in the female urethra. *Neurourol Urodyn* 2007;26:254–61.

5. Lose G, Colstrup H, Saksager K, Kristensen JK. New probe for measurement of related values of cross-sectional area and pressure in a biological tube. *Med Biol Eng Comput* 1986;24:488–925.

6. Ghoniem G, Stanford E, Kenton K, Achtari C, Goldberg R, Mascarenhas T, et al. Evaluation and outcome measures in the treatment of female urinary stress incontinence: International Urogynecological Association (IUGA) guidelines for research and clinical practice. *Int Urogynecol J Pelvic Floor Dysfunct* 2008;19:5–33.

9 Bladder diaries

Matthew Parsons

Introduction

The bladder diary is an important tool in the investigation of patients with lower urinary tract symptoms and voiding dysfunction, as there is poor correlation between subjective and charted estimates of diurnal and nocturnal urinary frequency.[1] There are different methods for recording information on voiding patterns. A frequency–volume chart is the simplest method and collects information on volumes voided and micturition times. A voiding or bladder diary provides a more detailed record. It facilitates history taking by acquiring information on incontinence episodes, pad usage and other information such as fluid intake, degree of urgency and degree of incontinence. Bladder diaries should be completed as part of the assessment before treatment and their use is recommended by the National Institute for Health and Clinical Excellence (NICE).[2]

Types of bladder diary

There are two methods for recording information in a bladder diary. The paper diary is the most common as it is easy to produce and store, inexpensive and convenient to post or hand directly to the patient (Figure 9.1). The alternative is an electronic bladder diary (Figure 9.2) such as the UroDiary™ (LifeTech, Stafford, Texas). This type of diary uses an intelligent character recognition programme and calculates a

Frequency Volume Chart

Time	Day 1 In	Day 1 Out	Day 1 Wet	Day 2 In	Day 2 Out	Day 2 Wet	Day 3 In	Day 3 Out	Day 3 Wet
7 am		340						260	
8 am	300			400	330		350		
9 am		200						170	
10 am	200	150		150	200		200		
11 am			W		175			150	
12 pm		200		150				50	
1 pm	150			150	200	W			
2 pm		175					320	200	
3 pm				200				200	
4 pm	450	150			220				W
5 pm		100					150		
6 pm		100	W	300			150	175	
7 pm	250	175		500	200/150				
8 pm	200	50		400	150/150	W	450	100	
9 pm	100				50	W		100	W
10 pm	350	180	BED	150			400	200	
11 pm					210	BED		210	BED
12 am									
1 am		270					200		
2 am	100					W			
3 am		300							
4 am					210				
5 am									
6 am									

Figure 9.1a An example of a frequency volume chart in a paper bladder diary

Frequency Volume Chart
IMPORTANT – PLEASE READ INSTRUCTIONS CAREFULLY

It is vitally important that you fill in the chart overleaf as accurately as possible over a three-day period prior to attending your test.

It is designed to help us take a closer look at your fluid intake and output, and leakage if any.

For each day, record *how much* (mls. if possible) and *what time* you drink and write it down in the *IN* column.

When you go to the toilet, *measure the urine* you pass using a jug (mls. if possible) and write it down in the *OUT* column.

If you *leak urine*, put a *W* in the *WET* column.

When you go to bed put a line on the chart next to the appropriate time. This allows us to see the difference between what is happening during the day and during the night.

FOR EXAMPLE:

Time	DAY 1		
	IN	OUT	WET
6 am			
7 am		350 mls	
8 am	150		
9 am		90	W
10 am	200		
11 am			W

Passed urine at 7.25 am – 350mls
Drank tea at 8.15 am – 150mls
Passed urine (90 mls) and leaked at 9.10 am
and so on

NB If it is difficult to fill in the full 5 days, PLEASE try and fill in at least two days, as this will greatly help us diagnose your condition.

Figure 9.1b Instructions for completing a paper bladder diary

centile ranking for results, correcting for age and 24-hour voided volume. The diaries are scanned into a computer and a customised report is generated.

Using a bladder diary

Women should be encouraged to complete a diary for a minimum of 3 days and should cover variations in their usual activities, such as both working and leisure days.[2] Non-completion of a diary does not exclude urinary symptoms.[3] Bladder diaries are especially useful to establish pattern and amount of fluid intake in the following circumstances:

- compulsive or excessive fluid consumption is easily identified. Metabolic disorders such as diabetes may be identified in this way
- normal fluid volumes consumed at inappropriate times (for example, at bedtime) may cause nocturia
- excessive intake of alcohol or caffeine causing exacerbation of symptoms.

Culture- and age-specific instructions should be included, explaining what information is to be collected and the relevance for the woman attending for investigation (Figure 9.1b).

Information provided by a bladder diary

The diary should have space to record fluid intake, with at least a recording of the volume and time of consumption. There should also be room to record the volume and timing of urine passed and a recording of any relevant lower urinary tract symptoms, especially incontinence (Figure 9.1a). The calculations on frequency and nocturia should conform to the International Continence Society's standardisation of terminology.[4] For the purposes of calculation, daytime frequency is defined as the number of voids during waking hours and includes the last void before going to bed. Nocturia is rising to void at night, preceded and followed by sleep, including the first void of the morning.[4] There is an underlying assumption, when calculating day and night volumes, that voiding occurs immediately after rising in the morning and before going to bed.

The information usually obtained from a simple bladder diary is:

- functional bladder capacity, which should be 300–500 ml
- frequency of diurnal and nocturnal micturition
- total voided volume during the day and during the night
- duration of day and night, to allow calculation of rate of production of urine
- a semi-objective evaluation of the severity of urinary incontinence and associated or provocative events.

Advantages of a bladder diary

Bladder diaries are more accurate than recall when recording urinary symptoms.[1] They are cheap and easy to use. They can guide many aspects of conservative treatment, especially timing and types of fluids. Bladder capacity has a strong relationship with age and 24-hour voided volume and is not absolute. Bladder diaries do not diagnose detrusor overactivity or stress urinary incontinence but they are the only way to diagnose nocturnal polyuria. Learned or habitual frequency may also be semi-objectively assessed.

Comparison of electronic and paper bladder diaries

Paper charts need to be manually calculated, which may be time consuming in a busy clinic, and inaccuracies may occur when pressed for time. Additionally, studies have shown a strong positive relationship between bladder capacity and 24-hour voided volume and a strong

(a)

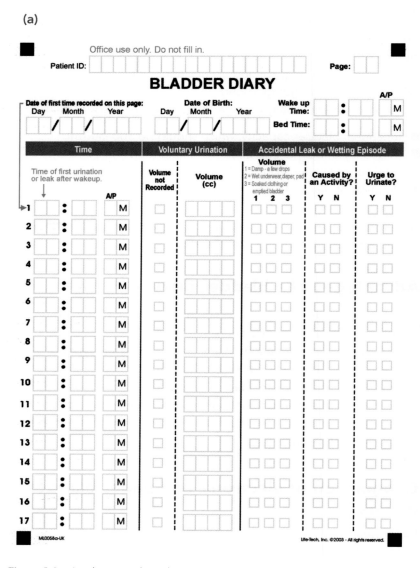

Figure 9.2a An electronic diary, the UroDiary™ chart

(b)

BLADDER DIARY INSTRUCTIONS

This confidential, computer-processed Bladder Diary will give your doctor important information about the times and amounts of your urinations and any accidental losses of urine that you may have. By filling out your Bladder Diary completely and accurately, you will contribute significantly to your medical care.

Please fill your Diary according to the following instructions:

1. Keep your Diary for _____ consecutive days.
2. Begin your Diary when you wake up on a day that you know you will be able to: (a) continue all remaining days without interruption and, (b) follow your usual sleep/wake pattern.
3. "Bed Time" is the time you turn the lights out in preparation for sleep.
4. On each line, record the time and information about either a voluntary urination or an accidental leak.
5. The first time recorded on each page must be on or after the wakeup time.
6. Use as many pages as needed to record all urinations or leaks from the time you wake up until you wake up the next morning. However, always begin a new page every time you wake up.
7. To record a voluntary urination, measure the amount of urine you pass in cubic centimeters (cc) and record in the "Volume (cc)" column. Use the measuring vessel provided in your Bladder Diary kit.
8. If you are in a place (e.g. restaurant) where you cannot measure your urine volume, just "X" the "Volume not Recorded" box and record the time of the urination.
9. In the accidental leak or wetting episode column, record how much you leaked, whether it was caused by an activity (e.g. running, jumping, lifting, walking, coughing), or if an urge to urinate caused you to wet before you could get to the toilet.
10. If you have any questions, call _____.

Marking Instructions

1. Use one of the soft lead pencils provided in your Bladder Diary Kit. If you lose these pencils you can substitute black ink or any No. 1 pencil. Please do not use blue ink.
2. Keep all entries inside the blue boxes
3. Enter "Xs" in the blue check boxes. Please do not use check marks.

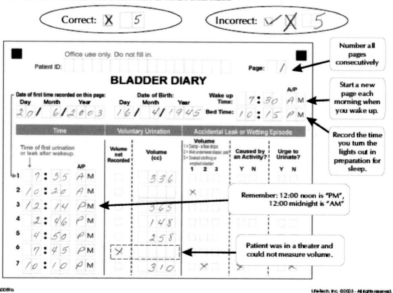

Figure 9.2b Electronic bladder diary instructions

negative relationship with age in normality and detrusor overactivity.[5,6] 'Eye-balling' paper charts, while widely practised, may therefore lead to inaccuracy.

Clinical cases

CASE 1

Bladder diary of a woman with urinary stress incontinence (Figure 9.3).

This 51-year-old woman presented with a history of stress urinary incontinence. Note that the diary shows a normal frequency – the absolute number is eight voids/day, which is on the 57th centile. Bladder capacity is only slightly below average. Forty percent of her incontinence episodes are associated with activity. She underwent subtracted cystometry and was diagnosed with urodynamic stress incontinence.

CASE 2

Bladder diary of a woman with detrusor overactivity (Figure 9.4).

This 59-year-old woman complained predominantly of urgency, frequency, and nocturia: the so-called 'overactive bladder' syndrome. Note the reduced bladder capacity and high frequency. This diary also confirms the nocturia, despite normal urine production rates. None of her leak episodes were associated with activity.

Compared with women who have stress incontinence, women with detrusor overactivity tend to have:[7]

■ higher voiding frequency

- lower volume/void, more urge-related than activity-related leaks
- smaller volume and equally frequent leaks
- more severe incontinence symptoms.

CASE 3

Clinical benefit of the bladder diary (Figure 9.5).

This 59-year-old woman was referred by her general practitioner with symptoms of overactive bladder. She did not leak urine. In line with NICE guidance, she completed a bladder diary, the results of which are shown in Figure 9.5a. It can be seen that she has quite a high fluid intake at 2.16 litres/day. She has relatively normal urine production rates and a normal night frequency. However, for her age and volume voided, her frequency is elevated and her bladder capacity reduced. She attended our nurse-led clinic, where she received fluid and lifestyle advice, as well as deferment techniques and support. The nurses used the diary report to illustrate and guide her in order to correct her fluids, in a manner similar to 'biofeedback'.

Four months later, her diary was repeated (Figure 9.5b). She has reduced her intake to 1.5 litres/day, is now voiding seven rather than nine times/day and has a bladder capacity on the 50th centile, which enables her to sleep through the night. She was delighted with the outcome.

BLADDER DIARY RESULTS

Patient:
Patient ID
Age:
Sex: F
Physician:

Calculation Parameters
Volumes prorated: Yes
Percentile calculation: Adjust for age and volume
Diary Duration (Hours) 46.2
Start Date   22/05/2011

Frequency-Volume Data

Per 24 Hours

	Amount	Percentile
Frequency (voids)	8.0	57%
Total Volume (ml)	2177	79%
Production Rate (ml/min)	1.51	78%

Volume Per Void (ml)

	Amount	Percentile
Minimum	100	68%
Maximum	550	38%
Average	297	61%
Range	450	22%

	Day		Night	
Day vs Night	Amount	Percentile	Amount	Percentile
Frequency (voids)	7.8	48%	0.0	75%
Total Volume (ml)	2177	93%	0	<1%
Production Rate (ml/min)	2.38	93%	0.00	<1%
Production Rate % of 24H	158%	>99%	0%	<1%

Incontinence Episodes

Average Episodes Per 24 Hours	0.8	Percent Caused by Activity	50%
Average Leak Size Score(Scale1-3)	1.0	Percent Accompanied by Urge	50%

Frequency-Volume Chart

Figure 9.3 Bladder diary of a woman with stress urinary incontinence

BLADDER DIARY RESULTS

Patient:
Patient ID
Age:
Sex: F
Physician:

Calculation Parameters
Volumes prorated: Yes
Percentile calculation: Adjust for age and volume
Diary Duration (Hours) 71.7
Start Date   07/06/2008

Frequency-Volume Data

Per 24 Hours	Amount	Percentile
Frequency (voids)	11.0	95%
Total Volume (ml)	2579	87%
Production Rate (ml/min)	1.79	85%

Volume Per Void (ml)	Amount	Percentile
Minimum	80	47%
Maximum	500	10%
Average	236	4%
Range	420	<1%

	Day		Night	
Day vs Night	Amount	Percentile	Amount	Percentile
Frequency (voids)	11.0	94%	0.0	47%
Total Volume (ml)	2270	93%	310	25%
Production Rate (ml/min)	2.16	89%	0.79	32%
Production Rate % of 24H	121%	75%	44%	8%

Incontinence Episodes

Average Episodes Per 24 Hours	1.1	Percent Caused by Activity	0%
Average Leak Size Score(Scale1-3)	1.0	Percent Accompanied by Urge	80%

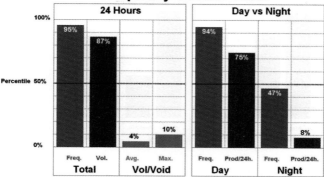

Figure 9.4 Bladder diary of a woman with detrusor overactivity

BLADDER DIARY RESULTS

Patient:
Patient ID
Age:
Sex: F
Physician:

Calculation Parameters
Volumes prorated: Yes
Percentile calculation: Adjust for age and volume
Diary Duration (Hours) 48.0
Start Date 23/03/2008

Frequency-Volume Data

Per 24 Hours	Amount	Percentile
Frequency (voids)	10.0	89%
Total Volume (ml)	2164	72%
Production Rate (ml/min)	1.50	72%

Volume Per Void (ml)	Amount	Percentile
Minimum	30	7%
Maximum	450	16%
Average	194	4%
Range	420	11%

	Day		Night	
Day vs Night	**Amount**	**Percentile**	**Amount**	**Percentile**
Frequency (voids)	9.0	90%	1.0	48%
Total Volume (ml)	1267	50%	897	97%
Production Rate (ml/min)	1.51	65%	1.49	83%
Production Rate % of 24H	101%	35%	99%	68%

Incontinence Episodes

Average Episodes Per 24 Hours	0.0	Percent Caused by Activity	0%
Average Leak Size Score(Scale1-3)	0.0	Percent Accompanied by Urge	0%

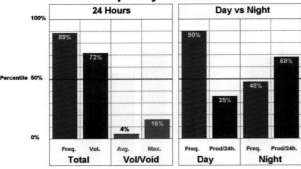

Figure 9.5a Bladder diary of a woman with symptoms of overactive bladder

BLADDER DIARY RESULTS

Patient:
Patient ID
Age:
Sex: F
Physician:

Calculation Parameters
Volumes prorated: Yes
  Percentile calculation: Adjust for age and volume
Diary Duration (Hours) 48.7
Start Date   12/07/2008

Frequency-Volume Data

Per 24 Hours	Amount	Percentile
Frequency (voids)	7.0	48%
Total Volume (ml)	1528	35%
Production Rate (ml/min)	1.06	35%

Volume Per Void (ml)	Amount	Percentile
Minimum	125	87%
Maximum	440	46%
Average	215	51%
Range	315	11%

Day vs Night	Day Amount	Day Percentile	Night Amount	Night Percentile
Frequency (voids)	6.9	63%	0.0	47%
Total Volume (ml)	1095	37%	433	42%
Production Rate (ml/min)	1.23	46%	0.79	27%
Production Rate % of 24H	116%	69%	75%	39%

Incontinence Episodes

Average Episodes Per 24 Hours	0.0	Percent Caused by Activity	0%
Average Leak Size Score(Scale1-3)	0.0	Percent Accompanied by Urge	0%

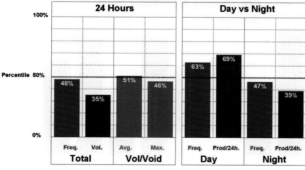

Figure 9.5b Bladder diary of the same woman 4 months later

111

BLADDER DIARY RESULTS

Patient:
Patient ID
Age:
Sex: F
Physician:

Calculation Parameters
Volumes prorated: Yes
  Percentile calculation: Adjust for age and volume
Diary Duration (Hours) 65.0
Start Date   09/07/2011

Frequency-Volume Data

Per 24 Hours	Amount	Percentile
Frequency (voids)	14.0	>99%
Total Volume (ml)	1319	51%
Production Rate (ml/min)	0.92	52%

Volume Per Void (ml)	Amount	Percentile
Minimum	20	11%
Maximum	105	<1%
Average	70	<1%
Range	85	<1%

Day vs Night	Day Amount	Day Percentile	Night Amount	Night Percentile
Frequency (voids)	9.6	98%	4.4	>99%
Total Volume (ml)	671	39%	648	78%
Production Rate (ml/min)	0.80	44%	1.08	71%
Production Rate % of 24H	87%	21%	117%	75%

Incontinence Episodes

Average Episodes Per 24 Hours	0.0	Percent Caused by Activity	0%
Average Leak Size Score(Scale1-3)	0.0	Percent Accompanied by Urge	0%

Frequency-Volume Chart

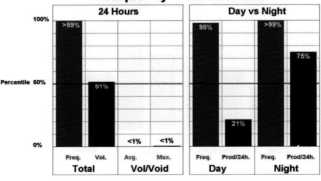

Figure 9.6 Bladder diary of an elderly woman with symptoms of overactive bladder and reduced bladder capacity

BLADDER DIARY RESULTS

Patient:
Patient ID
Age:
Sex: F
Physician:

Calculation Parameters
Volumes prorated: Yes
Percentile calculation: Adjust for age and volume
Diary Duration (Hours) 72.5
Start Date 09/07/2011

Frequency-Volume Data

Per 24 Hours	Amount	Percentile
Frequency (voids)	7.0	53%
Total Volume (ml)	1248	24%
Production Rate (ml/min)	0.87	24%

Volume Per Void (ml)	Amount	Percentile
Minimum	50	38%
Maximum	400	52%
Average	160	33%
Range	350	30%

Day vs Night	Day		Night	
	Amount	Percentile	Amount	Percentile
Frequency (voids)	5.6	47%	1.3	90%
Total Volume (ml)	645	14%	603	68%
Production Rate (ml/min)	0.66	13%	1.28	73%
Production Rate % of 24H	76%	4%	147%	>99%

Incontinence Episodes

Average Episodes Per 24 Hours	0.0	Percent Caused by Activity	0%
Average Leak Size Score(Scale1-3)	0.0	Percent Accompanied by Urge	0%

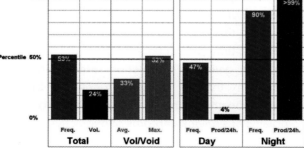

Frequency-Volume Chart

Figure 9.7 Bladder diary of an elderly woman with symptoms of overactive bladder and nocturnal polyuria

CASE 4

Bladder diary in the ageing population (Figure 9.6).

Nocturia occurs when the functional bladder capacity is exceeded by the volume of urine produced during sleep. This may occur because the functional bladder capacity is reduced as a result of ageing, or because the urine production rate is abnormally high at night (or a combination of the two).[8] As a rule of thumb, nocturnal urine production should be less than 35% of the 24-hour total[8] and, where this is exceeded, 'nocturnal polyuria' is said to occur. Other authors have used the night production rate to define it.[9]

In a study comparing night and day, using production rates corrected for age reduced the variability of the normal range by 40% and expressing the night production rate as a proportion of the 24-hour production rate reduced it by a further 20%.[10] It is important to identify nocturnal polyuria, as the treatment can be markedly different.

The diary of the 79-year-old woman shown in Figure 9.6 has a total voided volume of 1.17 litres. She has a daytime frequency of 8.3, which is above the 99th centile for her age and volume. However, with a night-time production of 306 ml, this is 26% of her 24-hour volume, giving a production rate on the 30th centile. The problem then is reduced functional bladder capacity, confirmed on the diary. The 82-year-old woman in Figure 9.7 complains of similar symptoms of overactive bladder. Her 24-hour volume is much larger and so is her night volume. This illustrates the importance of calculating as a proportion rather than relying on absolute values. Her night production is 1.01 litres but her maximum bladder capacity is 390 ml, so it stands to reason that she will void three times in the night. Her night volume is 42% of her 24-hour total, with a night production rate above the 99th centile. This woman has nocturnal polyuria, as well as a small bladder capacity for her volume.

LEARNING POINTS
- Bladder diaries are more accurate than recall when recording urinary symptoms.
- Bladder diaries should be completed as part of the assessment, before treatment.
- Bladder diaries are virtually the only method for diagnosing nocturnal polyuria.
- Use of a bladder diary for a minimum of 3 days, including a weekend, is recommended good practice.
- A bladder diary usually provides information on functional bladder capacity, daytime and nocturnal micturition, urinary output and a semi-objective assessment of severity of incontinence.
- Electronic bladder diaries are useful in generating a customised report and when analysing large numbers of figures in a research setting.

References

1. McCormack M, Infante-Rivard C, Schick E. Agreement between clinical methods of measurement of urinary frequency and functional bladder capacity. *Br J Urol* 1992;69:17–21.
2. National Collaborating Centre for Women's and Children's Health. *Urinary Incontinence: the Management of Urinary Incontinence in Women*. London: RCOG Press; 2006 [http://guidance.nice.org.uk/CG40].
3. Heit M, Brubaker L. Clinical correlates in patients not completing a voiding diary. *Int Urogynecol J Pelvic Floor Dysfunct* 1996;7:256–9.
4. Abrams P, Cardozo L, Fall M, Griffiths D, Rosier P, Ulmsten U, et al. The standardisation of terminology of lower urinary tract function: report from the Standardisation Sub-committee of the International Continence Society. *Neurourol Urodyn* 2002;21:167–78.

5. Amundsen CL, Parsons M, Tissot B, Cardozo L, Diokno A, Coats AC. Bladder diary measurements in asymptomatic females: functional bladder capacity, frequency and 24-hr volume. *Neurourol Urodyn* 2007;26:341–9.
6. Amundsen CL, Parsons M, Cardozo L, Vella M, Webster GD, Coats AC. Bladder diary volume per void measurements in detrusor overactivity. *J Urol* 2006;176:2530–4.
7. Parsons M, Amundsen CL, Vella M, Webster GD, Coats AC. Bladder diary patterns in detrusor overactivity and urodynamic stress incontinence. *Neurourol Urodyn* 2007;26:800–6.
8. Weiss JP, Blaivas JG. Nocturia. *J Urol* 2000;163:5–12.
9. Asplund R, Sundberg B, Bengtsson P. Desmopressin for the treatment of nocturnal polyuria in the elderly: a dose titration study. *Br J Urol* 1998;82:642–6.
10. Parsons M, Tissot W, Cardozo L, Diokno A, Amundsen CL, Coats AC. Normative bladder diary measurements: night versus day. *Neurourol Urodyn* 2007;26:465–73.

10 Pad testing

Emmanuel Karantanis

Introduction

Pad testing is most often used in the objective assessment of women with urinary incontinence. It involves the use of pre-weighed continence pads to capture urinary leakage over a period of time. The pads are then weighed to calculate the amount of leakage on completion of the test.

Why are pad tests performed?

Pad tests are most commonly used in the research setting:

- to provide objective confirmation of urinary incontinence before and after treatment
- to measure objectively the quantity of urine loss as a measure of severity: a 24-hour pad test loss of greater than 75 g represents severe incontinence in women with stress urinary incontinence[1]
- as a general aid when determining type of incontinence: women with pure stress urinary incontinence have been shown to leak less than 100 g in 24 hours and those with overactive bladder have more severe leakage;[1] however, there is significant overlap, such that pad tests cannot be used to make an accurate diagnosis
- to help to differentiate between urine and vaginal discharge in women who may have excessive vaginal fluid loss: urinary incontinence is unlikely if less than 2 g of loss is found on a

24-hour pad test;[2] such tests should not be conducted with panty liners, as they have a tendency to evaporate their fluid.

Types of pad test

There are several methods of pad testing which differ in duration of test, ranging between 1 hour and 72 hours, and in the activities undertaken during the test. The two most common methods used for pad testing are 1-hour and 24-hour tests.

One-hour pad testing

One-hour pad tests are performed in a clinical setting, under the supervision of a continence nurse or doctor. They include a filling phase, during which the woman spends 15 minutes drinking 500 ml of fluid. This is followed by a series of provocative manoeuvres, such as coughing and jumping, to try to stimulate urinary leakage. Pads are weighed before and at the end of the test. Pad loss greater than 1 g is designated as significant or a 'positive pad test'.

Twenty-four-hour pad testing

Twenty-four-hour tests are performed at home. Women are provided with a set of pads and advised not to modify their normal drinking or activities. The aim of such tests is to document leakage in a normal home environment.

Performing a pad test

Equipment

Only three components are needed to perform a pad test:

- pads
- snap-lock bags (one per test) to keep moisture in (all pad wrapping and adhesives should be placed in the bag to maintain an accurate post-test recording)
- weighing scales: scales accurate to 0.1 g should be used.

One-hour pad test

The ICS Standardisation Committee has set out a standard protocol for the 1-hour pad test.[3]

1. Test is started without the patient voiding.
2. Pre-weighed pad or collecting device is put in place by the subject and the first 1-hour test period begins.
3. Subject is given 500 ml sodium-free liquid to drink within a short period (maximum 15 minutes) and then sits or rests for 15 minutes.
4. Half-hour period: subject walks, including stair climbing equivalent to one flight up and down.
5. During the remaining period the subject performs the following activities:
   - (i) standing up from sitting, ten times
   - (ii) coughing vigorously, ten times
   - (iii) running on the spot, 1 minute
   - (iv) bending to pick up small object from floor, five times
   - (v) wash hands in running water, 1 minute.
6. At the end of the 1-hour test, the pad or collecting device is removed and weighed.

7. If the test is regarded as representative, the subject is asked to void and the voided volume is recorded.
8. If the test is not regarded as representative, the test is repeated, preferably without voiding.

24-hour pad test

The 24-hour pad test has not been standardised. The following is a description of the 24-hour pad test as used by the author.

1. Women are provided with five incontinence pads (such as Tena Lady Normal™, SCA Hygiene Products, Göteborg, Sweden; these pads are less evaporative than panty liners, less absorptive than thicker pads and more accurately reflect the fluid deposited on them).
2. Each pad is pre-weighed within a snap-lock bag. Women start the test is started in the morning and change to a new pad every 4 hours during the day. At the end of the day, they wear their final pad for about 8 hours overnight and complete the test upon waking.
3. The pads are returned within 7 days, as they are shown to hold moisture if sealed.[4] Whenever a pad is removed, it must be reinserted in the original snap-lock bag with wrappings and adhesives that were originally weighed.
4. Women do not need to undertake any particular provocative activities apart from their usual activities. It is useful to perform any vigorous activities that usually produce leakage activities while undertaking the test.
5. Twenty-four-hour pad tests are particularly informative when performed simultaneously with a bladder chart.

Comparison of 1-hour and 24-hour pad tests

Twenty-four-hour pad tests have been found to be repeatable and more sensitive than 1-hour pad tests.[4] They require fewer staff resources and less time and have been correlated with subjective severity measures.[5,6] The upper limit of normal for a 24-hour pad test is 2 g when using Tena Lady Normal™ pads.

Summary

Pad tests are of most value in the research setting before and after treatment, as an objective endpoint of urinary incontinence. The activity undertaken by the women during a test may influence the results such that a similar level of activity should be performed when pad testing for comparison before and after treatment. Women's compliance with 24-hour pad tests decreases once cured. The same types of pads should be used for all patients before and after treatment, as pads have different absorptive and evaporative qualities. The major limitation of the pad test is the lack of diagnostic ability.

Learning points

- Pad tests are most commonly used in the research setting as an objective endpoint of urinary incontinence.
- Pad test methodology varies in duration and type of activities undertaken, with 1-hour and 24-hour tests being the most common types.
- The same type of pad should be used throughout and Tena Lady Normal™ pads are the most suitable absorptive type.
- A positive 1-hour pad test is urine loss greater than 1 g and a positive 24-hour test is a loss greater than 2 g.

References

1. O'Sullivan R, Karantanis E, Stevermuer TL, Allen W, Moore KH. Definition of mild, moderate and severe incontinence on the 24-hour pad test. *BJOG* 2004;111:859–62.
2. Karantanis E, O'Sullivan R, Moore KH. The 24-hour pad test in continent women and men: normal values and cyclical alterations. *BJOG* 2003;110:567–71.
3. Abrams P, Blaivas JG, Stanton S, Andersen JT. The standardisation of terminology of lower urinary tract function. *Neurourol Urodyn* 1988;7:403–26.
4. Versi E, Orrego G, Hardy E, Seddon G, Smith P, Anand D. Evaluation of the home pad test in the investigation of female urinary incontinence. *Br J Obstet Gynaecol* 1996;103:162–7.
5. Karantanis E, Allen W, Stevermeuer TL, Simons AM, O'Sullivan R, Moore KH. The repeatability of the 24-hour pad test. *Int Urogynecol J Pelvic Floor Dysfunct* 2006;16:63–8.
6. Lose G, Jorgensen L, Thunedborg P. 24-hour home pad weighing test versus one-hour ward test in the assessment of mild stress incontinence. *Acta Obstet Gynecol Scand* 1989;68:211–15.

11 Pre-test assessment using questionnaires

Ramandeep Basra, Nikki Cotterill, Swati Jha, Cornelius J Kelleher and Stephen Radley

Why use quality of life questionnaires?

Lower urinary tract symptoms cause significant health-related quality of life impairment for sufferers.[1] In clinical practice, a physician's assessment of the disease burden is inaccurate and non-reproducible and physicians often underestimate the impact of lower urinary tract symptoms on patients' quality of life.[2] Patients report higher subjective distress in questionnaires than structured interviews.[2] To optimise the management of symptoms, it is important that their impact is assessed in a meaningful manner.

Lower urinary tract symptoms and their impact can be measured in several ways; however, the only validated way of measuring the patient's perspective is through the use of psychometrically robust self-completion questionnaires.[1] Questionnaires should only be used if they provide a valid, reproducible, rapid assessment of patient-reported disease impact, which can elicit symptom impact and which is also useful for the evaluation of treatment efficacy.[1]

The King's Health Questionnaire

Features

The King's Health Questionnaire (KHQ) is a condition-specific, self-completion questionnaire (Table 11.1).[3] It was developed and validated following six pilot studies. These studies demonstrated good validity and reliability.[3] The KHQ has been extensively used in pharmaceutical clinical studies.

Table 11.1 Format of the King's Health Questionnaire

Part	Content
1	General health perception (GHP)
	Incontinence impact (II)
2	Role limitations (RL)
	Emotions
	Sleep/energy
	Severity (coping) measures
	Physical limitations (PL)
	Social limitations (SL)
	Personal relationships (PR)
3	Urinary symptoms bother scale

The National Institute for Health and Clinical Excellence (NICE) has recommended use of the KHQ in the assessment of women with lower urinary tract symptoms.[4] The questionnaire has a grade A recommendation (based on level 1 evidence: systematic reviews and meta-analyses of randomised trials) for use in research and clinical practice for the assessment of health-related quality of life in adult men and women with lower urinary tract symptoms.[1]

The KHQ has been adopted by the International Consultation on Incontinence (ICI) modular questionnaire as one of the core quality-of-life assessments for patients with lower urinary tract dysfunction (ICIq LUTS QoL).[5] There are over 39 linguistic validations of the scale, making it an ideal instrument for multinational studies. Completion time for the questionnaire is 10–15 minutes. The KHQ measures nine domains of quality of life: general health perception, incontinence impact, social limitations, role limitations, physical limitations, personal relationships, severity measures (coping strategies), sleep/energy and emotions. There is also a ten-item symptom severity scale. Each domain of the questionnaire has an individual score (maximum score 100); a greater value indicates increased impact on quality of life (with the exception of the general health perception domain).

Minimal important difference (MID) is the degree of change in each domain score of the KHQ which indicates a meaningful improvement in quality of life to the patient. The MID distinguishes between 'noise' and meaningful improvement. MID analysis of the KHQ revealed that a five-point change in KHQ domain score represented a small change in health-related quality of life and a 10–15-point change represented a moderate change.[6]

Quality-adjusted life years (QALYs) provide a measure of the value of health outcomes and are used in the economic evaluation of health interventions. A QALY is the arithmetic product of life expectancy and a measure of the quality of the remaining life years. QALY calculations based on the KHQ have been published, which make it ideal for inclusion in studies where health economic analyses are important.[7]

A six-item short form of the KHQ has been developed. This questionnaire consists of two domains: limitation of daily life and mental health.[8]

Advantages and disadvantages of using the KHQ

Advantages

- Rapid and concise assessment of symptoms and 'bother'.
- Useful adjunct to clinical assessment of patients with lower urinary tract symptoms.
- Useful for evaluating the effectiveness of treatment or an intervention.
- Allows patients to bring to light symptoms that they may be too embarrassed to mention during the clinical consultation.
- Measures patients' perception of lower urinary tract dysfunction.
- Inexpensive method of data collection.
- Useful tool for clinical audit and research.

Disadvantages

- Questionnaires completed by proxy by a carer or partner may be inaccurate.
- Structured questionnaires do not allow patients to provide additional information.
- Response to postal questionnaires may be poor.
- Bias in completing questionnaires:
  - 'faking good' to please the clinician or to conform with socially accepted values
  - 'faking bad' to emphasise the severity of the condition
  - 'end aversion': the reluctance to use the extreme categories of a scale.
- Difficulty understanding spoken or written English limits completion (but linguistic validations available).
- Incomplete completion (deliberate or unintentional).
- Confounding factors, such as recent life events, may affect patient responses to questions.

How to access the KHQ

Copies of the KHQ (and scoring system) are available from:

- NICE guideline CG40 *Urinary Incontinence: the management of urinary incontinence in women.* Urinary incontinence: implementation advice appendix: King's Health Questionnaire [www.nice.org.uk/CG40].
- ICI Modular Questionnaire website (with permissions) [www.iciq.net/ICIQ.LUTSqolmodule.html].
- ProQolid: Patient-Reported Outcome and Quality of life Instruments Database. King's Health questionnaire [http://proqolid.org/instruments/king_s_health_questionnaire_khq].

ePAQ: electronic personal assessment questionnaire

The electronic personal assessment questionnaire to measure, process and present pelvic floor symptoms and their impact on quality of life (ePAQ-PF) was originally derived from paper-based instruments (the Birmingham Bowel and Urinary Symptoms Questionnaire and the Sheffield Prolapse Questionnaire).[9–11]

Features of ePAQ-PF

The standard one-item-per-page format includes stem questions relating to symptom frequency and sub-questions relating to impact (Figure 11.1). It is a reliable and valid measure of urinary, bowel, vaginal and sexual symptoms, with 19 psychometrically robust, clinically meaningful domains, scored from 0 (indicating best) to 100 (worst health status).[12–14]

Individual items are scored on a four-point scale and summative domain scores are transformed to a scale of 0–100. ePAQ's urinary

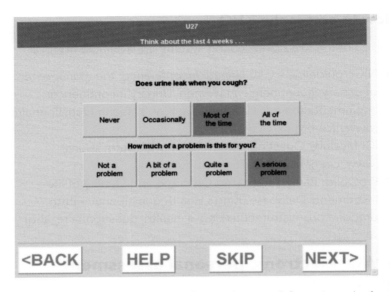

Figure 11.1 The standard screen format of an ePAQ item with four-point scales for symptom frequency and bother. Sub-questions on bother are only shown when symptoms are present. The toolbar at the bottom of eachscreen allows navigation through the questionnaire as well as access to specific help pages. A touchscreen or mouse may be used to complete the questionnaire

dimension provides scores for stress urinary incontinence, overactive bladder, voiding, pain and quality of life (Figure 11.2). The impact of interventions on pelvic floor symptoms as well as sexual function and quality of life can therefore be readily be monitored (Figure 11.3).[15]

The simple interactive format of ePAQ (including help pages and automatic skipping of irrelevant items) supports unsupervised self-completion. Levels of missing data are low and satisfaction ratings from patients high. Clinical assessment is crucial to the diagnosis of most pelvic floor conditions, although their sensitive nature means that disclosure is often incomplete or inaccurate. Most patients report enhanced communication with ePAQ, in the context of both hospital

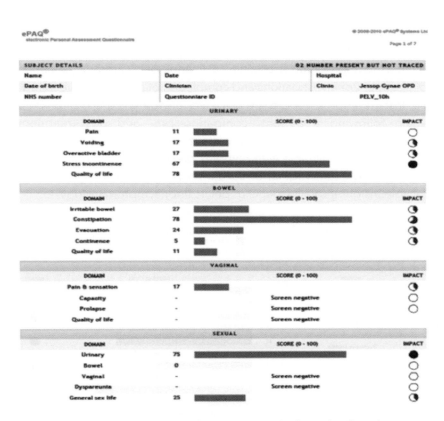

Figure 11.2 ePAQ summary report: domain scores in the four pelvic floor dimensions are shown both numerically and graphically, with clockface icons to the right-hand side showing the maximum bother associated with the symptoms contributing to that domain

and virtual clinic appointments. Pelvic floor medicine is particularly demanding of well-designed measures of symptoms and quality of life, particularly as there is such overlap between different elements of the multidisciplinary service, including urogynaecology, colorectal surgery, reconstructive urology, physiotherapy and nursing, in both primary and secondary care.

Online ePAQ completion followed by telephone consultations form the basis of the Virtual Urogynaecology Clinic, allowing triage of patients to appropriate specialties, exchange of information, initiation of treatment or investigations and completion of post-operative follow-up. Instant progress reports are provided for women completing ePAQ again following treatment, comparing pre- and post-treatment symptom scores as well as a global impression of change (Figure 11.3).

ePAQ is also valuable with complex presentations, with coexistent urinary, colorectal, vaginal or sexual problems, providing valid and reliable insight into all aspects of pelvic floor symptomatology.

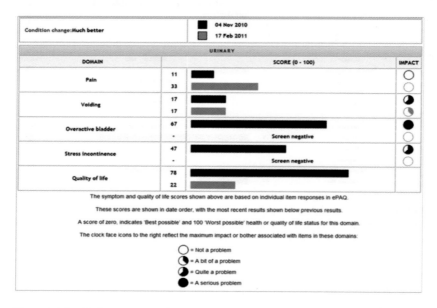

Figure 11.3 ePAQ progress report: ePAQ was completed by this patient at initial consultation and again 3 months following intravesical botulinum A injection therapy for overactive bladder. Follow-up was conducted in the Virtual Clinic (ePAQ on-line plus telephone consultation). Global rating of change is shown on the top left-hand side of the report. These reports may also be included in discharge summaries and correspondence with GPs

How to access ePAQ-Pelvic Floor

ePAQ Systems Ltd was one of the first NHS spin-out technology companies to be created. Information about using ePAQ may be obtained from www.epaq.co.uk.

International Consultation on Incontinence Modular Questionnaire

Features

The International Consultation on Incontinence Modular Questionnaire (ICIQ) was developed to provide a universally applicable, standardised series of self-completion assessment instruments to evaluate lower urinary symptoms, lower bowel symptoms and vaginal symptoms.[16,17] It consists of a collection of 14 high-quality questionnaires.[17] Separate modules need to be completed for bowel, bladder, prolapse and sexual dysfunction.

ICIQ can be used in men and women irrespective of age, with varied causes for their symptoms, facilitating the use of common questionnaires in many patient groups. It was developed from a standard protocol for the development and translation of ICIQ questionnaires. The content of the questionnaires is derived from patients and clinical experts, providing a robust evidence base for inclusion.

Core modules evaluate the core symptoms of lower pelvic dysfunction, namely lower urinary tract, lower bowel and vaginal symptoms. Additional specialised and detailed modules are available, such as overactive bladder symptoms, nocturia, quality of life and sexual matters (Table 11.2).

The ICIQ is an international collaborative project encouraging worldwide standardisation of assessment and is available in numerous languages.

Table 11.2 The International Consultation on Incontinence Modular
Questionnaire structure

CONDITION	MODULES	
	RECOMMENDED	OPTIONAL
A: Core modules		
Urinary symptoms	Males: ICIQ-MLUTS Females: ICIQ-FLUTS	Males: ICIQ-MLUTS LF Females: ICIQ-FLUTS LF
Vaginal symptoms and sexual matters	ICIQ-VS	
Bowel symptoms	ICIQ-B	
Urinary incontinence	ICIQ-UI Short Form	ICIQ-UI LF*
B: Specific patient groups		
Nocturia	ICIQ-N	
Overactive bladder	ICIQ-OAB	
Neurogenic	ICIQ-Spinal Cord Disease*	
Long-term catheter users	ICIQ-LTC*	
Children	ICIQ-CLUTS*	

* Developmental modules

How to access the ICIQ questionnaires

Questionnaire modules are supplied free of charge for clinical practice
and academic research. They can be accessed via the project website:
www.iciq.net.

Table 11.2 continued.

RECOMMENDED ADD-ON MODULES			
QoL	Generic QoL	Sexual matters	Post-treatment
ICIQ-LUTSqol	SF-12	Males: ICIQ-MLUTSsex Females: ICIQ-FLUTSsex	
ICIQ-VSqol*	SF-12		ICIQ-Satisfaction*
ICIQBSqol*	SF-12	Males: ICIQ-Bsex* Females: ICIQ-Bsex*	
ICIQ-LUTSqol	SF-12	Males: ICIQ-MLUTSsex Females: ICIQ-FLUTSsex	
ICIQ-Nqol	SF-12	Males: ICIQ-MLUTSsex Females: ICIQ-FLUTSsex	ICIQ-Satisfaction*
ICIQ-OABqol	SF-12	Males: ICIQ-MLUTSsex Females: ICIQ-FLUTSsex	
	SF-12		
ICIQ-CLUTSqol*			

References

1. Abrams P, Cardozo L, Khoury S, Wein A, editors. *Incontinence, Volume 1. Basics and Evaluation. 3rd International Consultation on Incontinence June 2004.* Edition 2005. Co-sponsored by International Continence Society and Société Internationale d'Urologie. Plymouth: Health Publications; 2005.
2. Rodriguez LV, Blander DS, Dorey F, Raz S, Zimmen P. Discrepancy in patient and physician perception of patient's quality of life related to urinary symptoms. *Urology* 2003;62:49–53.

3. Kelleher CJ, Cardozo L, Khullar V, Salvatore S. A new questionnaire to assess the quality of life of urinary incontinent women. *Br J Obstet Gynaecol* 1997;104:1374.

4. National Collaborating Centre for Women's and Children's Health. *Urinary Incontinence: The Management of Urinary Incontinence in Women*. National Institute for Health and Clinical Excellence Guideline CG40. London: RCOG Press; 2006 [http://guidance.nice.org.uk/CG40/Guidance/pdf/English].

5. International Consultation on Incontinence Modular Questionnaire website (with permissions) www.iciq.net/ICIQ.LUTSqolmodule.html.

6. Kelleher CJ, Pleil AM, Reese PR, Burgess SM, Brodish PH. How much is enough and who says so? *BJOG* 2004;111:605–12.

7. Brazier J, Czoski-Murray C, Roberts J, Brown M, Symonds T, Kelleher C. Estimation of a preference-based index from a condition-specific measure: the King's Health Questionnaire. *Med Decis Making* 2008;28:113–26.

8. Homma Y, Uemura S. Use of the short form of King's Health Questionnaire to measure quality of life in patients with an overactive bladder. *BJU Int* 2004;93:1009–13.

9. Bradshaw HD, Hiller L, Farkas AG, Radley S, Radley SC. Development and psychometric testing of a symptom index for pelvic organ prolapse. *J Obstet Gynaecol* 2006;26:241–52.

10. Hiller L, Radley S, Mann CH, Radley SC, Begum G, Pretlove SJ, et al. Development and validation of a questionnaire for the assessment of bowel and lower urinary tract symptoms in women. *BJOG* 2002;109:413–23.

11. Jackson S, Donovan J, Brookes S, Eckford S, Swithinbank L, Abrams P. The Bristol Female Lower Urinary Tract Symptoms questionnaire: development and psychometric testing. *Br J Urol* 1966;77:805.

12. Radley SC, Jones GL, Tanguy EA, Stevens VG, Nelson C, Mathers NJ. Computer interviewing in urogynaecology: concept, development and psychometric testing of an electronic pelvic floor assessment questionnaire in primary and secondary care. *BJOG* 2006;113:231–8.

13. Jones GL, Radley SC, Lumb J, Jha S. Electronic pelvic floor symptoms assessment: tests of data quality of ePAQ-PF. *Int Urogynecol J Pelvic Floor Dysfunct* 2008;19:1337–47.

14. Jones GL, Radley SC, Lumb J, Farkas A. Responsiveness of the electronic Personal Assessment Questionnaire-Pelvic Floor (ePAQ-PF). *Int Urogynecol J Pelvic Floor Dysfunct* 2009;20:557–64.

15. Jha S, Radley S, Farkas A, Jones G. The impact of TVT on sexual function. *Int Urogynecol J Pelvic Floor Dysfunct* 2009;20:165–9.

16. Abrams P, Avery K, Gardener N, Donovan J. The international consultation on incontinence modular questionnaire: www.iciq.net. *J Urol* 2006;175:1063–6.

17. Staskin D, Kelleher C, Avery K, Bosch R, Cotterill N, Coyne K, et al. Patient-reported outcome assessment. In: Abrams P, Cardozo L, Khoury S, Wein A, editors. *Incontinence: Proceedings of the fourth International Consultation on Incontinence, July 5–8, 2008*. 4th ed. Plymouth: Health Publication Ltd; 2009. p. 363–412.

12 Ultrasound as a tool in urodynamics

Demetri C Panayi and Vik Khullar

Introduction

Ultrasound of the bladder is commonly used in clinical practice as a non-invasive estimate of bladder volume when assessing post-void urinary residual. The advantages of ultrasound as a technique are that it is non-invasive, risk free and is easily applied and accessible when compared with traditional techniques, which are comparatively time consuming, invasive and involve exposure of the patient to X-rays.

Equipment

Two types of ultrasound equipment are available:

- dedicated bladder scanner: a mechanical sector probe to calculate a volume (although this may pick up artefact: any fluid-filled structure such as postnatal lochia or ovarian cyst)
- standard linear array transabdominal or transvaginal ultrasound: this estimates volume using an equation – height (cm) x width (cm) x depth/0.7 (cm). Estimated volume is unreliable at higher volumes because of a non-linear increase as urinary volume increases.

Indications for ultrasound in urodynamics

Bladder volume

Ultrasound can be used to measure bladder volume; for example, estimation of residual volume.

Urethral hypermobility

Ultrasound of the bladder neck can be used to assess urethral hypermobility (Figure 12.1). Increased bladder neck mobility is associated with stress urinary incontinence and can be measured ultrasonically using an X–Y coordinate system. The position of the bladder neck in terms of rotational angle and descent of the bladder neck can be determined (Figure 12.1). This method has a specificity of 83.1% and positive predictive value of 67.6% for urodynamic stress incontinence.[1] The urethral angle (α angle) is more accurate and specific, with a higher positive predictive rate than the angle between the proximal and distal urethra (β angle).[2]

Urethral sphincter volume

Using three-dimensional ultrasound, the volume of the urethral sphincter can be measured (Figure 12.2) and this technique has been validated.[3]

Advanced ultrasound techniques

Measurement of bladder wall thickness

Measurement of the thickness of the bladder wall has been validated using the transvaginal, transperineal, translabial or transabdominal

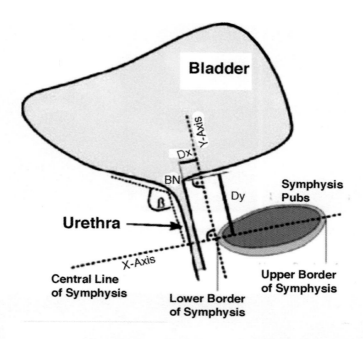

Figure 12.1 The X axis is a horizontal line through the symphysis pubis and the Y axis is a line perpendicular to the X axis, allowing measurement of certain parameters. Here, Dy is the perpendicular distance from the X axis to the bladder neck

approach. The scan is carried out after voiding, with a bladder volume of less than 50 ml. Parasagittal measurements are taken at the trigone, the anterior wall and the dome of the bladder (Figure 12.3).

This technique is not often used in clinical practice but a mean measurement greater than 5 mm is associated with (but not diagnostic of) detrusor overactivity.[4] This relationship may be lost if the integrity of the urethral sphincter is compromised, such as in women with mixed incontinence.

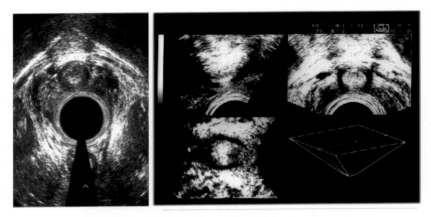

Figure 12.2 Measuring the volume of the urethral sphincter

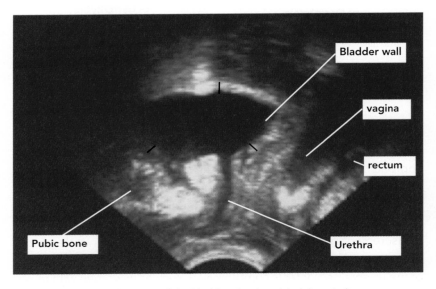

Figure 12.3 A sagittal section of the bladder; the three black lines indicate measurement of the bladder wall

Ultrasound and assessment of the pelvic floor

The application of ultrasound in the assessment of lower urinary tract and pelvic floor conditions is growing. The advent of three-dimensional ultrasound has allowed closer evaluation of anatomical structures believed to be associated with female urinary incontinence. While urodynamics remains the mainstay of objective assessment of symptoms described by women, ultrasound is likely to be used increasingly to provide the anatomical parameters in conjunction with

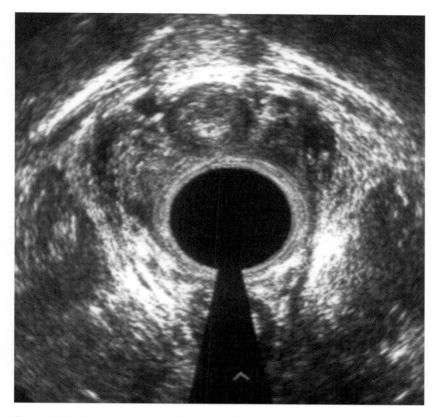

Figure 12.4 Transvaginal image of the pelvic floor

functional parameters provided by urodynamics. Two-dimensional and three-dimensional ultrasound have been employed to statically and dynamically image the pelvic floor.[5,6] The application of ultrasound in the identification of levator injury is currently being used as a research tool (Figure 12.4).

LEARNING POINTS

■ Residual urine volume can be estimated with linear array ultrasound using the formula height (cm) x width (cm) x depth/0.7 (cm).

■ Bladder scanners will estimate the volume of any underlying fluid-filled structure.

■ Ultrasound of the bladder neck can be used to assess bladder neck hypermobility, with 83% specificity, although it is not always predictive of stress incontinence.

■ Ultrasound is currently being used in research to estimate bladder wall thickness and levator injuries.

References

1. Chen GD, Su TH, Lin LY. Applicability of perineal sonography in anatomical evaluation of bladder neck in women with and without genuine stress incontinence. *J Clin Ultrasound* 1997;25:189–94.
2. Pregazzi R, Sartore A, Bortoli P, Grimaldi E, Troiano L, Guaschino S. Perineal ultrasound evaluation of urethral angle and bladder neck mobility in women with stress urinary incontinence. *BJOG* 2002;109:821–7.
3. Toozs-Hobson P, Khullar V, Cardozo L. Three-dimensional ultrasound: a novel technique for investigating the urethral sphincter in the third trimester of pregnancy. *Ultrasound Obstet Gynecol* 2001;17:421–4.
4. Khullar V, Cardozo LD, Salvatore S, Hill S. Ultrasound: a noninvasive screening test for detrusor overactivity. *Br J Obstet Gynaecol* 1996;103:904–8.
5. Dietz HP, Steensma AB. The prevalence of major abnormalities of the levator ani in urogynaecological patients. *BJOG* 2006;113:225–30.
6. Dietz HP, Shek KL. Levator defects can be detected by 2D translabial ultrasound. *Int Urogynecol J Pelvic Floor Dysfunct* 2009;20:807–11.

Index

abdominal (rectal/vaginal) catheters 8, 9

abdominal leak-point pressure (ALPP) 92–3, 95

abdominal pressure (p_{abd})
  baseline 36, 37
  cough response 37–8, 39
  impaired transmission 85, 86
  sudden changes 85, 87

accommodation, poor 44, 45

air-filled catheters 9
  calibration 17
  setting up 12
  zeroing 16

ambulatory urodynamic monitoring (AUM) 67–79
  advantages and disadvantages 76–7
  annotation during 74
  clinical cases 77–8
  conventional cystometry vs 67–8
  equipment 69–72
  indications 68
  interpretation and analysis 74–5
  patient information 73
  performance 68
  troubleshooting 75

anaphylactoid reactions, contrast media 61

artefacts 81–90
  checking for 37–8, 39, 88
  cystometry 84–8
  pressure flow 89
  uroflowmetry 24, 25, 26, 82–4

bladder capacity see functional

bladder capacity; maximum cystometric capacity

bladder diaries 99–115
  advantages 103
  ambulatory urodynamics 70, 71
  clinical cases 106–15
  completion 102
  electronic vs paper 103–6
  information provided 102–3
  types 99–102

bladder diverticulae 59, 60, 63

bladder herniation 59, 61

bladder neck mobility, assessment 136, 137

bladder trabeculation 60, 63

bladder volume, measurement 136

bladder wall thickness, measurement 136–7, 138

calibration, equipment 16–17, 18

commode 6

compliance, bladder 42
  high 44
  low (poor) 42–4, 45, 47, 48

contrast medium, iodine-based 55, 61

cough tests
  during bladder filling 41, 43
  checking for artefacts 37–8, 39, 88
  detrusor overactivity 51–2
  urodynamic stress incontinence 46–7, 58

cystocele 62

cystometry/cystometrogram 35–52
  abnormal detrusor function 42–5
  ambulatory urodynamics vs 67–8

artefacts 84–8
clinical cases 47–51
equipment 7–10
factors influencing measurements
    81–2
filling 40–7, 91–3
machine calibration 17, 18
normal detrusor function 41–2,
    43
patient preparation 2–3
patient sensations 40, 41
performance 36–41
post-test care 47
pre-test tests 35–6
quality checks 37–8, 39, 88
setting up equipment 11–16
urethral function testing 91–3
urodynamic stress incontinence
    46–7
voiding 47, 58, 93

detrusor leak-point pressure 92
detrusor overactivity
    ambulatory urodynamics 74, 77–8
    bladder diary 106–7, 109
    cystometrogram 44–5, 48–9,
        51–2
    provocative manoeuvres 45, 46,
        51–2
    videocystourethrography 58
detrusor pressure (p$_{det}$)
    baseline 36, 37
    cough responses 37–8, 39
    normal profile 41–2, 43
detrusor sphincter dyssynergia 59
dome covers 10
double-lumen catheters 8

elderly women, bladder diaries
    114–15
electronic bladder diaries 99–102,
    103–6
electronic personal assessment
    questionnaire: pelvic floor (ePAQ-PF)
    127–31

equipment 5–19
    ambulatory urodynamics 69–71
    calibration 16–17, 18
    pad testing 119
    setting up 11–16
    ultrasound 135
    videocystourethrography 55,
        56–7

filling catheters 8, 9
filling rate, cystometry 40
first desire to void 41, 42
flowmeters 5, 6
    calibration 17
    types 5, 21
flow patterns 24–32
flow rate testing see uroflowmetry
fluid-filled catheters 8
fluid-filled cystometry systems
    calibration 17, 18
    equipment 7–8, 10
    setting up 11, 12, 13, 14
    zeroing 15, 16
fluid intake 102
fluoroscopy 55, 56–7, 58
frequency, urinary
    bladder diaries 106–7, 109–15
    defined 102–3
frequency-volume chart 99, 100–1
functional bladder capacity
    measurement 103
    reduced 114–15

gravimetric flow rate measurement 21

indications for urodynamic testing 1–2
intermittent flow 24, 26, 31–2
International Consultation on
    Incontinence Modular Questionnaire
    (ICIQ) 131–3
        LUTS QoL module 124, 127, 133
        modules 132–3
intravesical pressure (p$_{ves}$)
    baseline 36, 37
    cough response 37–8, 39

gradual rise 85, 87
impaired transmission 85, 86
sudden changes 85, 87

King's Health Questionnaire (KHQ)
124–7

laboratory, urodynamics 5
Liverpool nomograms 23

manometer tubing 10
maximum cystometric capacity 41, 42
maximum flow rate (Q_{max}) 23
    artefacts 24, 25, 26
    reduced 24, 26, 27, 29
    several peaks 24, 31
    very high 24, 32
    voided volume and 22–3, 28, 29
Medicines and Healthcare products
    Regulatory Agency 10
minimal important difference (MID)
    125
mixed urinary incontinence,
    stress-predominant 64
movement, patient 82, 83

National Institute for Health and
    Clinical Excellence (NICE) 1, 99,
    124, 127
neurological disease
    uroflowmetry 26–7
    videocystourethrography 59
nocturia
    clinical case 112–13, 114–15
    defined 103
    value of bladder diaries 102
nocturnal polyuria 114–15

one-hour pad test 118, 119–20, 121
overactive bladder
    bladder diaries 106–7, 109–15
    cystometrogram 48, 49
    pad testing 117

pad testing 117–21

1-hour vs 24-hour 121
indications 117
methods 118
performance 119–20
pelvic floor, ultrasound assessment
    139–40
performance of tests 2
position, patient
    cystometrogram 40
    provoking detrusor overactivity
        45
    urodynamic stress incontinence
        46
post-void residual urine volume (PVR)
    elevated 26, 27, 31–2
    measurement 22, 35, 136, 140
    normal 42
preparation, patient 2–3
pressure flow artefacts 89
pre-test questionnaires 123–32
prolapse, pelvic organ
    clinical cases 31–2, 62
    reduction 47, 93
ProQolid 127
provocative manoeuvres
    cystometry 45, 46, 51–2
    one-hour pad test 118, 119
    videocystourethrography 55–8
    see also cough tests

Q_{max} see maximum flow rate
quality-adjusted life years (QALY) 125
quality of life questionnaires 123–31
questionnaires, pre-test 123–32

rectal (abdominal) catheters 8, 9
rectal contractions 75, 76, 85, 88
residual urine see post-void residual
    urine volume
rotating disc flowmeters 5, 21

sensations, patient, during bladder
    filling 40, 41
single-lumen catheters 8
Siroky nomograms 23

solid-state cystometry systems
  ambulatory monitoring 71–2
  calibration 17
  equipment 8–9, 10
  setting up 12
  zeroing 16
straining, abdominal 24, 27, 31–2, 83
stress incontinence, urinary
  bladder diary 103, 106, 108
  classification 58–9
  pad testing 117
  ultrasound evaluation 136
  videocystourethrography 64
  see also urodynamic stress
    incontinence
stress tests see provocative
  manoeuvres
supervoiders 24, 32
suprapubic tapping 26–7

temperature, cystometry infusate 40
twenty four-hour pad test 118, 120, 121

ultrasound 135–40
  advanced techniques 136–40
  equipment 135
  indications 136
urethral function tests 91–6
  advantages 95
  filling cystometry 91–3
  indications 95
  limitations 95–6
  specific 93–6
  voiding cystometry 93
urethral hypermobility, assessment
  136, 137
urethral pressure profilometry (UPP)
  93, 94
urethral pressure reflectometry (UPR)
  94
urethral retro-resistance pressure
  (URP) 94
urethral sphincter
  female, continence mechanism
    91, 92

volume measurement 136, 138
urethral strictures 24, 29–31
urethrotomy 29–31
urgency
  during bladder filling 41
  detrusor overactivity 48, 49
urinary stress incontinence see stress
  incontinence, urinary
urinary tract infections, testing 36
UroDiary™ 99
urodynamic stress incontinence
  ambulatory urodynamics 78
  cystometrogram 46–7, 50
  grading 58
  see also stress incontinence,
    urinary
uroflowmetry 21–33
  artefacts 24, 25, 26, 82–4
  clinical cases 29–32
  equipment 5–6
  men with voiding symptoms 26
  parameters assessed 22–3
  patterns of flow 24–7
  performance 22
  preparation for 22
  setting up 11
  women with incontinence 26

vaginal (abdominal) catheters 8, 9
vesical leak-point pressure 92
vesicoureteric reflux 59, 63
videocystourethrography (VCU) 55–65
  advantages 58–9
  clinical cases 62–4
  conduct 55–8
  equipment and facilities 55, 56–7
  imaging 58
  limitations 61
voided volume 22–3, 28
  effects on Q_{max} 22–3, 28, 29
voiding diaries see bladder diaries

zero pressure, setting 14–16, 17, 18
  errors 84, 85